ENTERING THE WORLD
The De-Medicalization of Childbirth

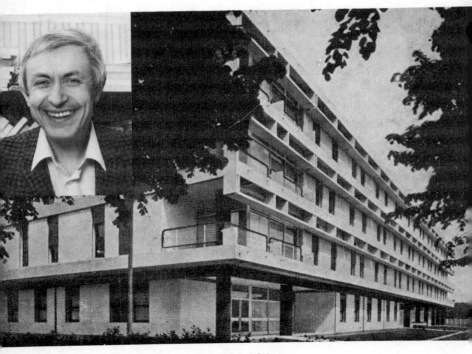

The general hospital in Pithiviers, France. Inset Michel Odent

CONTENTS

Note to the English Edition
Publishers' Note
An Introduction   9
    Dora Henschel, Senior Midwifery Tutor,
    King's College Hospital, London

A Tribute to Michel Odent   15
    Murray W. Enkin, MD, FRCS (C)
    Dept. of Obstetrics and Gynaecology,
    McMaster University, Hamilton, Ontario

Foreword   19

PART ONE: Ideas
    Chapter One – The Expropriation of Birth   25
    Chapter Two – Waiting for Leboyer   31
    Chapter Three – Who Preceded Leboyer?   34
    Chapter Four – Feeling and Reason   42
    Chapter Five – Love and Civilization   60

PART TWO: Experience
    Chapter Six – In the Beginning   73
    Chapter Seven – Preparation for Birth   79
    Chapter Eight – A Change?   90
    Chapter Nine – The People Who Came to Us   99
    Chapter Ten – Discussions and Deliberations   112
    Chapter Eleven – Scepticism and Criticism   132
    Chapter Twelve – A Call for Militancy   151
Recommended Reading   155
A Glossary for Laymen   157

'Consign your books to the fire. And you will soon be forgotten, Monsieur Leboyer.'
FRANCOISE TOURNIER

'Birth without violence was a marvellous poem to the glory of life and the joy of living, the birth of an evident truth . . .'
ROGER GENTIS

'Foolish the doctor who despises the knowledge acquired by the ancients.'
HIPPOCRATES

'Speak, thou that art the elder, for it becometh thee, but with sound judgment; and hinder not music.'
ECCLESIASTICUS, 32:3.

Note to the English Edition

This book was first published in France in 1976. One of my aims at that time was to point out the necessity of taking collective militant action against all institutionalized violence in general, and of changing the usual conditions of birth in particular. It was not until the famous London Birthrights Rally on 4 April 1982 that the first collective action of any dimensions took place. On that day I also met Marion Boyars and together we planned a translation of this book. This was more than just a coincidence.

Media coverage has brought the maternity unit at Pithiviers to a much wider public in the English-speaking world today. As a result we are constantly being asked about our background and development. This book (brought up-to-date from the 1976 edition) is an answer to many of those questions. We have made great leaps forward. *Bien Naitre* was inspired by the simultaneous publication of Ivan Illich's *Medical Nemesis* (new edition published in Britain as *Limits to Medicine: Medical Nemesis, The Expropriation of Health*) and Frederick Leboyer's *Birth Without Violence*. The appearance of these two works brought about the most daring and the most fruitful of our periods of progress, in terms of our thinking, our emotional responses and our daily practice.

Michel Odent

Publishers' Note

As this translation from the French is intended for American and British readers, a clarification of the term 'midwife' may be useful:

In France, most accredited midwives enter their profession directly (rarely with a previous nursing degree) and qualify after a three-year training period in state-run schools of midwifery.

In the United States, qualified nurses are trained and certificated, generally after one year's training. There is a strong movement in the United States to induct more accredited midwives.

In Britain, state registered nurses become certificated midwives after an additional eighteeen-month training period in a school of midwifery. Direct entry – which is rare – requries a three-year training course.

As most midwives in all three countries have some nurse's training in addition to their speciality, the book frequently adopts the designation 'nurse-midwife'.

An Introduction
Dora Henschel

It is a great privilege to write the foreword to the English translation of Doctor Michel Odent's first book. The thoughts and considerations molding his work represent a unique contribution to the practice of midwifery and obstetrics.

The book lends perspective to our understanding of an approach to childbirth that is positive and allows the woman freedom. Here trust replaces fear, and the baby is welcomed into the world as a uniquely sensitive human being.

Doctor Odent practices in the maternity unit of the public hospital in Pithiviers, France. For those not familiar with his background the following brief notes may provide a useful introduction.

I was introduced to Doctor Odent and his maternity unit by one of the former students of our nurse-midwifery training school. I had eagerly accepted an invitation when I learned that Frederick Leboyer's ideas of non-violent birth were practised there. Reading his book *Birth Without Violence* had originally left me with a certain resentment: it criticizes relentlessly the unfeeling care and handling of the newborn baby by nurse-midwives and doctors. Nonetheless, I had occasionally wondered whether true gentleness of touch and the reduction of sensory stimulation immediately after birth would really alter a baby's usual behavior.

Despite the later and perhaps more spectacular

developments I was to watch at two subsequent visits, it was the first visit which left the deepest impression.

I found that in the maternity unit in Pithiviers the birth process was expected to be normal. This very positive approach pervaded the whole atmosphere. The nurse-midwives were certainly alert to any deviation from the normal, but it was not conveyed to the mother. At the same time they and Doctor Odent watched the woman's instinctive reactions during labor and from these observations changes developed in the pattern of care.

As a result at each of my three visits to Pithiviers, I have seen an evolution of approaches to pain relief and to birth.

On admission of the woman in labor a general and obstetric examination was made by the nurse-midwife. Assessment of the progress of labor and its effect on both mother and fetus were made as necessary. If all was well she had full freedom of movement.

During my first visit this applied only to the first stage of labor. The baby was born with the mother on a conventional labor ward bed. Yet it was the birth I had come to see – the incredible experience of 'Birth without Violence'. The lights were dimmed, little was said except quietly spoken words of encouragement, a record played soft music, the only other sound apart from the woman's effort during a contraction and her breathing. During the birth the nurse-midwife neither supported the perineum nor controlled the emergence of the baby's head.

After feeling for the cord, and with another push, the midwife lifted the baby gently on to the mother's abdomen, soft and warm from the recent effort. To my surprise no fierce cries pierced the tranquillity of the room. The baby breathed quietly, had good color and tone and slowly seemed to wake as if from a dream. Some babies showed they wanted to suckle; in others this urge seemed delayed until later. To watch the serene expression on their faces as they opened their eyes and surveyed their new world was something new for me, as was the lack of fuss and commotion, the peace and joy, and the utter simplicity of the birth process. It was not just the Leboyer approach I witnessed. This birth experience was giving tremendous satisfaction. I was assured that the events of the five labors and births I had seen were quite usual. But if a labor had to end in a vacuum extraction (6%) or a Caesarian section (5%) Leboyer's principles of caring for the newborn were considered even more important.

Of course, the baby's condition would be ascertained at birth and all life-saving methods would be used when necessary!

On my second visit the 'Salle Sauvage' (birthing room) had been initiated. The dark brown walls and the subdued light and the vast double bed with its brightly colored cushions created a non-medical environment.

During labor the bed might be used for her to rest on, she was given freedom of movement, no particular position was imposed, and she was comfortable. However, the bed was not used much. The women preferred to be up and about, especially during a contraction. They liked leaning forward with their arms around their partner's neck, often moving their hips back and forth or in a circular motion.

To my utter astonishment most of them stayed on their feet during the second stage and for the delivery. During the contraction they were either supported from behind or by two people, one on each side. This position, the supported squat, kept the trunk straight, while the knees were bent. The nurse-midwife knelt in front of the mother and 'caught' the baby. The mother then sat on a thick disposable sheet on the floor, massaged and held her baby. Leboyer's approach to the birth was still part of the care. The bath was placed between her legs, and it was the mother who could bathe her baby, still attached by the cord to the placenta.

When I visited Pithiviers for the third time I found that Doctor Odent had been giving much thought to the discovery of endorphins – the body's own mechanism for pain relief. It was the time when he introduced an age-old medium which induces comfort and relaxation – a pool with warm water in which the woman would spend much of her time in labor. In an already peaceful environment the water seemed to help her reach a level of consciousness where pain was less intense. Added to this the cervix dilated faster and occasionally it happened that the baby was actually born under water – without ill effect.

Not all women sought this medium. The others pre-ferred the 'Salle Sauvage' though not the bed. Most other births now took place with the mother in the supported squatting position, rather than lying down. Today this is called 'Active Birth'.

The book explains the philosophy and psychology which make such births possible – yet they are not enough. The personnel of a unit, the conditions and the physical environment must be right to put them into practise. I found these to be very different to maternity units in this country.

The midwives rarely change. Only six midwives staff the unit for between 900-1000 deliveries a year. They work in pairs, 48 hours on duty followed by four days off. Their work is chiefly concerned with women in labor and birth. They also give some post-natal care. Ante-natally, the women are seen and examined by Doctor Odent. All other duties were carried out by one other grade of staff, the Aides Soignantes. Their work combined that of our domestics, nursing auxiliaries, and nursery nurses. They work in the department, three at a time, for eight-hour shifts, covering the 24 hours.

This very simple and practical arrangement of staffing is unthinkable in our units. And it is this lack of hierarchical arrangement which prevents conflict. There is equality not only between members of staff, but also between staff and mothers and babies – everyone matters equally. Such a positive atmosphere allows freedom and does not tolerate restrictions. The considerable experience of the professionals can allow this freedom to be expressed. The wishes of the women are respected and they need have no fear that routine technical interference will be imposed on them. As a result they accept it when it *has* to be used, because the course of labor or the condition of the fetus has become abnormal.

The main reason why this maternity unit had developed in such a different direction from others became clear to me very early during my first visit. Doctor Odent is not an obstetrician with the usual background we would expect in England. Approximately 17 years earlier he had been appointed surgeon to the hospital, to find himself called for any obstetric complications and emergencies which occurred in the maternity unit. At that time, this situation was not unusual in France, where obstetrics was still the Cinderella of medical practice. Ambitious young doctors were unlikely to choose this field for a promising career. For any doctor in this situation the lack of an obstetric background would prove a challenge and a daunting task to conquer. This apparent disadvantage materialized into a very positive advantage. To the skills of the surgeon, Doctor Odent soon added the skills required for abnormal obstetrics, although forceps were relegated to the 'museum of ancient torture instruments'! The art and science of obstetrics were learned from practical experience with the help of the midwives, from reading widely on the subject, and from talking and listening to the needs of the women. Searching more widely than just for the physical aspects of health, Doctor Odent, with an open mind relatively uncluttered by conventional obstetrics, gradually directed the development of the unit towards a holistic approach and philosophy of obstetrics.

The physical well-being of the mother, fetus and baby became part of a much wider concept of total health, where mental and emotional fulfilment was also essential. The combination of philosopher and psychologist in an obstetrician is all too rare. Mothers and babies owe him a great debt for putting his advanced thinking into practice.

Dora Henschel

A Tribute to Michel Odent
Murray W. Enkin

I was glad to be given the opportunity to write an appreciation of this book. In it, Michel Odent says many of the things that I would like to say, in ways that I could not say them. We are all products of our environments, of the influences which impinge upon us. We react in different ways, to different inputs. It is exciting to see how often we reach similar conclusions by such disparate pathways.

Insights, both scientific and transcendental, are recognized only when we are ready to receive them. How many keen observers recognized the cause of childbed fever before Semmelweis? How many wise women knew the role of fear and tension in childbirth pain before Grantly Dick Read? How many loving people felt with and for newborn babies long before Frederick Leboyer?

Leboyer wrote a beautiful book, a gentle book, a sensitive book, full of love, poetry and pictures. It was a book that struck a responsive chord in mothers and others who were ready to listen. He expounded a philosophy of love. He wrote about feelings he had learned about by feeling himself. He relived the pain of his own birth. Whether that reliving was real or fancied is irrelevant. As only a poet can, he expressed the hurt and pain and love he felt in a way that helped many of his readers feel that same pain and hurt and love. He described how the pain and hurt might be minimized and the love be realized.

We are slow, however, to recognize poets in our society. We are overawed and overwhelmed by our technology. Like all aspects of our lives today, birth is enveloped by a variety of technical rituals. In modern hospitals, even those practising so-called family centred maternity care, procedures take precedence over the deeper feelings of mother and baby. Many professionals – and many mothers as well – have looked on Leboyer as yet another technique to be included in their armamentarium. If this were true, as such the 'Leboyer technique' could and should be looked on and evaluated as should any intervention. Its objectives should be explicitly stated and it should be evaluated by properly controlled clinical trials. Far too few of the many interventions we use in the hope of somehow improving our reproductive outcome have been subjected to such trials. When trials have been carried out, the results have often been far different than expected. Shaving the pubic hair, for example, does not in fact decrease the risk of infection; enemas neither expedite labor nor prevent contamination of a sterile field. Electronic fetal monitoring has not been shown to lessen the risk of perinatal mortality in any of the 5 studies reported to the present time. And a meticulously controlled randomized clinical trial of the 'Leboyer technique' – dim light, delayed clamping of the cord, a warm bath for the newborn – carried out in our own unit at McMaster (Nelson et al., *New England Journal of Medicine*, 302,655-660, 1980) failed to show any benefit to either mother or baby over a gentle birth under more conventional conditions. We were disappointed but not surprised.

Doctor Leboyer was neither surprised nor disappointed in our results. I can still see his gentle smile as he admonished me: "You study too much. You should not study, you should feel.'

As a result of our scientific enquiry, born out of scepticism, we have rejected a technique and embraced a philosophy of family autonomy within a high-risk obstetrical care centre. Women have with them the companion or companions of their choice during both labor and delivery. Delivery rooms are used only when required; normally, birth takes place in a comfortable labor room. To the extent that they themselves desire, mother and family assume responsibility for the care of their new family member from the moment of birth, with help and guidance from the professional staff. Family centred care is looked on as an attitude rather than a protocol. Birth is recognized as a vital life event rather than a medical procedure.

Michel Odent and his colleagues in Pithiviers chose to follow a different direction. They neither studied nor practiced the 'Leboyer technique'. They listened to Leboyer, they listened to the mothers giving birth and to the babies born in their community. They realized that the things that really count cannot be counted, and simply put the principles of gentle birth into practice in the way that was right for them and for the women who came to them for care. Only later did they look to other fields of enquiry to justify their approach.

Many years ago John Seldon Miller (*Childbirth*, Atheneum, New York, 1963) wrote 'The present trend in our American way of life is towards total anaesthesia from the cradle to the grave. The infant, who is bottle-fed so she won't have to work for dinner, is surrounded by a superfluity of gadgets and toys that stifle all imagination ... When she gets pregnant she goes to her doctor who assures her that her life need not change in any way. This experience too will be sterile, automated, painless and emotionless. This is a vicious circle, exaggerated perhaps, but basically true. The events leading to the cradle offer one logical place to break this circle.'

Twenty years later, we are close to the apocalypse. Intuitively, we know that somehow, some way, we must change our direction. It may be too late. But it may not be too late. With expressive clarity, Dr. Odent has pin-pointed the place where we must start: 'It is among the dominant that we must first work to redevelop the ability to love'.

Doctor Odent has put his love, his faith and his principles into practice. It is time for us all to do the same.

Murray W. Enkin

FOREWORD

Early in 1974 Frederick Leboyer posed the following
question in his book *Birth Without Violence,* which was to
become a best-seller:

> Could it not be that birth is as painful for the child as
> giving birth once was for the mother?
> And if it is, does anyone care?

At the same time, in the English-speaking medical press
and in a French article, Ivan Illich introduced the concept
of medical nemesis which he was later to develop in a
book of that title. Nemesis, goddess of vengeance,
represents the divine force which descends on anyone
who had infringed the prerogatives of the divine. After
their struggle against the elements and against the slavery
imposed on them by other members of their own species,
human beings are now confronted by a third menace: the
threat of enslavement to their present gods, their tools.
Behind *Medical Nemesis (Limits to Medicine)* lies the
fundamental question: where is the proper dividing line
between what people can do for themselves or with the
help of friends and family, and what they require
professional help for?

Both Leboyer and Illich have seen their work described
as shocking. Both have inflamed much of the medical
establishment. We have found that the questions they ask
have led to a useful consideration of the conditions of
birth in industrialized countries. What ideas have we had?

How have they influenced our own lines of argument?
What effect have they had on our day-to-day practice?
These are the questions we attempt to answer in this
book.

The significance of Ivan Illich's work is that he has constructed a political critique of technology, to recognize the
point at which tools become tyrants rather than servants,
when institutions do more harm than good; in short, he
has defined the convivial society. He has focussed his
attacks on the inevitable implications of industrial society
world-wide, of transport, of academic and medical institutions.

In his analysis of the medical establishment, Illich has
sought to condemn the expropriation of health by exploring the various supposed aims of the healing professions:
the suppression of pain, the eradication of disease and
the struggle against death. He has examined the
medicalization of old age and death in some detail.

Our aim is to pursue the work of Illich with a consideration of the conditions of birth in industrialized countries,
using the 'Leboyer phenomenon' as a focus for discussion.

Leboyer has brought to light a clash of views which we
intend to examine. As a poet-obstetrician he has written of
and acted on feelings and emotions. Our intention is to
work from feeling through to rational argument which will
both direct, and be directed by, day-to-day practice.

We have been privileged to observe the 'Leboyer
phenomenon', to recognize the sometimes indifferent,
sometimes hostile, sometimes contemptuous, sometimes
superficial reception granted him in obstetric circles.

We have met Leboyer and observed him at work.

We have met couples at their wit's end and have shown them what birth can be by means of Leboyer's book and film and through personal or reported evidence.

We have met women whose desire to be mothers had been awakened by reading Leboyer's message.

We have attended meetings, conferences and screenings of the film *Birth* in a wide variety of contexts.

And, above all, we have gained food for thought from the everyday work in a maternity unit where the concept of birth without violence has profoundly changed the climate of opinion.

Experience has led our staff to a mass of divergent and apparently haphazard conclusions, many of them unexpected and difficult to classify. The variety and importance of the questions raised will help us to reveal the true significance of Leboyer's poetry.

Our immediate objective is to interpret Leboyer's words for those who find his oracular means of expression irritating or are hostile to poetry as a form of communication. We address ourselves particularly to the obstetrical technician.

Is a practical application possible? Is there not a danger that in so doing we shall erase or obscure what is essentially a subjective experience? Surely Leboyer has already said it all, in the simplest possible language:

There must be love
Without love you will be merely skilful.

If we presume to present a new reading of Leboyer, it is because our maternity unit is probably the only one where birth without violence has been rapidly assimilated into an institution, if it is ever possible to institutionalize an atmosphere. Also, having seen the perinatal mortality rate fall to 10 in 1000, we are convinced that we are travelling along the right road.[1]

---

[1]When the first edition of this book was published in 1976, the perinatal mortality rate in France was around 20 in 1000 (perinatal mortality being taken to mean after 180 days in the womb and before seven days of life).

Part One
IDEAS

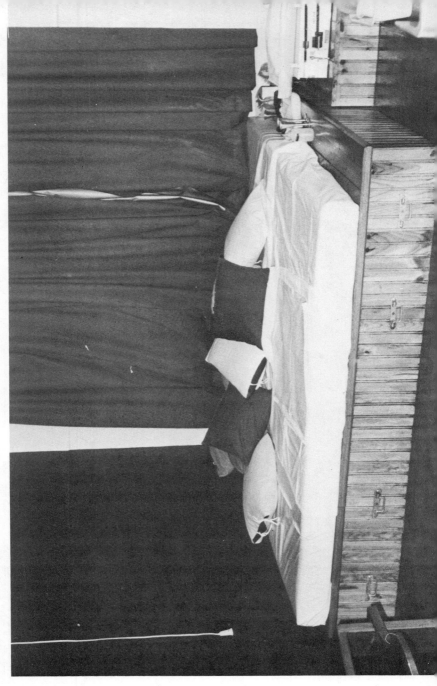

The birthing room ('salle sauvage')

Chapter One
THE EXPROPRIATION OF BIRTH

'Custom hides from us the true face of things.'
MONTAIGNE

It is our intention to describe our own experience of de-medicalization and the arguments for it, to present the reasons which led us to concentrate on birth rather than on labor, and to consider some of the further thinking our experience has provoked. But, before doing this, it may be useful to define what we see as the usual conditions of birth in industrialized countries.

In Holland, where home delivery is common, there are exceptionally low figures for perinatal morbidity and mortality which argue seriously in favor of home birth. Indeed, the family environment would appear to offer the best means of preventing many forms of dystocia (prolonged or painful labor due to insufficient contractions rather than anatomical abnormality), of de-medicalizing birth and of breaking down the technical barriers which frequently come between mother and child. However, it is generally accepted that the hospital environment provides maximum safety, as one can only talk about normal labor in the past, never in the future. Certainly the development of easily portable and reliable means of monitoring could facilitate a return to home birth, just as the treatment of chronic renal failure by the use of artificial kidneys has ceased to involve a stay in hospital. In fact, at the present time, most births in Britain, France and the United States take place in maternity units or obstetric departments, i.e. in state- or privately-run hospitals.

Maternity units are run by obstetricians who specialize in gynaecology *and* obstetrics, which means that they have chosen to concentrate, vocationally and professionally, on the woman more than the child. Most gynaecologist-obstetricians are male. Other specialists are becoming increasingly involved in the work of maternity units, particularly anaesthetists. Some make no secret of their intention to 'invade' the delivery room. Of course, there are also professional nurse-midwives, but as a general rule they have to obey instructions laid down by the head of department, and in private sector units they will often summon a doctor towards the end of labor. Recently some midwives have become aware of their oppression and their inferior status within a male-dominated medical power-structure. These women anticipate that obstetrics will become the battle ground for future political conflict. Obstetricians tend to see their role as being solely to ensure that the baby passes from the intra-amniotic to the aerial environment in the best possible thermodynamic conditions, with the least possible damage to the vital organs, particularly the brain.

Very few obstetricians stop to wonder which of their own acts or attitudes might impede the establishment of good parent-child relations; very few are aware of the fundamental importance of the very first child-object relation (with the maternal breast and the mother); very few stress the specific part fathers play at birth in regulating the mother-child relation and in symbolically separating the two; above all, very few obstetricians are aware of the way in which the ability to mother, to love, is transmitted from generation to generation, since the process by which a woman learns how to mother her children begins at her own birth. This limited view of their role explains why

obstetricians, or many of them, follow the delivery procedure that they now do.

It goes without saying that labor itself takes place in a
wide variety of conditions:

– not all women come to labor equal because they have
not been equally traumatized or equally well prepared
since childhood by their own mothers and their own
cultural background;

– not all women are equal because only a minority have
joined classes or groups which have helped them to
experience labor in a positive way;

– while material backgrounds may be much more
standardized, personal human environments remain
infinitely diverse;

– very few professionals know how to eliminate those
factors which inhibit the change in consciousness and the
fluctuations in hormonal balance necessary for the
physiological process of delivery. These factors include
light, rigid adherence to particular positions, fixed concentration on the vulva, and so on;

– analgesia frequently depends on pharmacological
methods (whether by general or local anaesthesia), or
sometimes on acupuncture, hypnosis and sophrological
technique.

Monitoring of delivery may be purely clinical, but it is
generally agreed that the continuity and reliability
achieved with electronic monitoring offer the best
guarantees in many cases. (By electronic monitoring we
mean both the continuous recording of physical
parameters, such as uterine contractions and fetal
heartbeat, and the periodic measurement of biological
parameters such as blood chemistry from a drop of blood
taken from the fetal scalp. Uterine contractions and fetal

heartbeat are recorded by external electrodes placed on the woman's abdomen; only after the membranes have broken is it possible to use internal tocographs and fetal scalp electrodes.)

The conditions of birth, on the other hand, appear to be fixed. Most commonly a technician wearing mask, cap, boots and gloves presides over the final stage of 'expulsion'. He stands in front of the woman who lies some distance from the ground, 'delivers' the baby's head with both hands, after an episiotomy where considered necessary, carefully examines the baby in bright lighting, then delivers the shoulders. As soon as the child is born its gender is announced, and immediately the mouth and nostrils are aspirated with a probe. The cord is quickly sectioned between two clamps and the baby laid on its back on a resuscitation table warmed by lamps. There is further aspiration, this time of the oesophagus and the tracheo-oesophagal fork so that the doctor can ensure that there is no occlusion of the oesophagus which will require surgery. An initial clinical examination calculates the Apgar[1] score and eliminates the possibility of gross malformation. The establishment of respiratory and cardiac rhythms is checked by stethoscope. The stump of the cord is dressed. In many western countries it is still common, or even obligatory, to administer an antiseptic eyewash.

Sometimes the baby is shown to its mother before it is weighed and dressed. At best it may be placed for a few

[1]The Apgar score, which is measured 1 minute and 5 minutes after birth, evaluates heart rate, respiration, muscle tone, reflexes and skin color. Each child can therefore be assigned scores between 1-10 from the moment of birth. There are advantages to this marking system in that it provides a code which can be understood by hospital staff and neo-natalogists, but we do have misgivings about including the Apgar score on official health records made out for individuals.

moments on her belly. Often the crying child will be given to her already swaddled. Generally there is no opportunity for the baby to manifest the archaic primary reflexes which exist in all healthy newborn infants, in particular the rooting reflex which enables the baby to search for, find and suck at its mother's breast a few minutes after birth. The extraordinary sensitivity of the newborn to smells, which is probably their way of identifying the mother at an early stage, is persistently disregarded in delivery rooms.

During its stay in the maternity unit care of the newborn baby is carried out either by or under the supervision of professionals. Indeed, some hospitals have taken things to such extremes that post partum monitoring involves greater separation of mother from child. The mother will be monitored by electrocardiography (in some cases even by arterial probes), while the baby is placed for two hours in an automatic incubator which registers skin temperature, fetal electrocardiogram and respiratory rhythm. An alarm system warns staff of the slightest anomaly. It is no exaggeration to speak of total erotic neutralization of the body from birth onward.

Although it is possible to outline a schema of the usual conditions of normal birth in the maternity units of technologically advanced countries, we should point out that 'normal' birth is becoming increasingly rare. Frequent recourse to epidural, and, even by some practitioners, general anaesthesia goes hand in hand with figures for instrumental extraction, usually by forceps, which may exceed 50%; while the percentage of caesarians is continually increasing throughout the western world. It could be argued that certain factors of acute fetal distress are attributable to high-technology maternity units, or at least to the particular way modern means of monitoring are being used. The use of external receptors, for example, involves prolonged lying on the back which tends to press the relaxed pregnant uterus against the lower vena cava. Ultrasound is often used to monitor fetal heartbeat. It is known, however, that ultrasound can cause lesions in living tissue by transforming sonic energy into thermal energy and by the mechanical effect responsible for cavitation. Even so, when ultrasound is used in obstetrics it is generally agreed to be harmless. Telemetric monitoring by radio waves has not entered current practice, and so far it continues to involve all the disadvantages of premature rupture of the membranes. The anxiety-inducing spectacle and atmosphere of present day delivery rooms may produce alterations in sympathetic muscle tone and the collapse of adrenergic reactions. All these influences may unite to produce what amounts to a 'dorsal decubitus' syndrome, a kind of postural shock, which is dangerous for the baby. In certain American hospitals, over 20% of births are artificially induced (Babson and Benson).

There appears to be no limit to the mechanical invasion of the delivery room. The American T. J. Kriewall (*University of Michigan News*, March 1975) has actually put the finishing touches to a prototype 'dilatometer' which suppresses vaginal touch, records cervical dilation and translates into computer language the energy expended by the laboring woman with the help of a small magnet fixed to one side of the cervix and a small magnetic feeler attached to the opposite side!

Will the obstetrician of tomorrow be sitting in front of a computer terminal screen?

Chapter Two
WAITING FOR LEBOYER

The fact that we are now able to describe our own experience of birth without violence is due to a series, or a coming-together, of random events. It is also true to say that when Leboyer's book appeared the climate in our own hospital was particularly well-suited to receive it.

We had been influenced for a dozen years or so by psychoprophylaxis, or rather a particular view of psychoprophylaxis. (What is sometimes known as the Lamaze method is a very limited and unsubtle interpretation of psychoprophylaxis.) We saw it as a weapon against that resignation to pain which turns the reproductive life of women into unmitigated torture. We also saw it as an approach to the important problem of mother-daughter relations which influence the whole structuring of femininity, since good preparation can help women better to determine their own position in relation to their mothers. By working against the picture of woman as object and victim, psychoprophylaxis has helped to remove passive methods of analgesia. It has always avoided drugs, general and local anaesthesia and epidurals in particular. Wherever the initial project of psychoprophylaxis has been understood, these passive methods have been seen as ways to alienate women through pain and to compound this alienation by emphasizing the evermore medicalized nature of birth. In several cases we have observed the negative effects of traditional ante-natal education which prepared the woman exclusively for labor, with a concentration on the woman herself. The chief concern as she came to term was to maintain control over her contractions. Labor was deemed successful when an active woman had stylishly rid her uterus of its passive contents, much as if she were emptying her bowels. Pulling faces and crying out were frowned upon. At its extreme, labor was experienced as an initiation test, not as the bringing forth of a child, and satisfactory behavior was regarded as a way of pleasing and thanking the staff. One useful innovation was the setting up of small groups of three pregnant women at most (sometimes only one woman could come) to meet together and to be introduced to all members of the staff individually.

The idea of planned parenthood had long since been welcomed within our hospital itself. A permanent family planning clinic had been set up there before the arrival of the official planned parenthood centre. Increased integration had gradually been achieved between family planning staff and maternity staff. Similarly, there were no rigid dividing lines between the maternity and the general surgery departments. Despite this, or because of it, the tendency to de-medicalize birth had grown stronger from one year to the next. The nurse-midwife was given much more responsibility; fathers were frequently present; induction, acceleration and active management of labor and the use of instruments became the exception.

We had developed specific practices, such as delayed cord-cutting and the avoidance of bright lights, but only as *modi operandi*, not as part of an overall considered system. From time to time statistical studies had been compiled to evaluate the effects of changes in staff and equipment and of technical innovations. For example, in 1972 the results of one line of research were published in a thesis[1] and showed a significant reduction in perinatal mortality over a ten year period:

overall perinatal mortality had dropped from 29 to 17 per 1000;
still births had dropped from 15 to 12 per 1000;
early neo-natal mortality dropped from 14 to 5 per 1000.

This study highlighted the part played by one particular conception of obstetrical psychoprophylaxis, if only in increasing contact between pregnant women and maternity staff, and the importance of widespread publicity about contraceptive methods in preventing large families. We should stress that this study preceded the introduction of electronic monitoring of labor.

These purely statistical studies were in no way incompatible with some preliminary thoughts about the many roles of nurse-midwife and obstetrician. We were already asking questions about the effects of the conditions of birth on the establishment of parent-child relations. We were already concerned about the extreme medicalization of birth. But we sometimes felt as though we were working and developing in isolation.

---

[1](M. Fesneau, *Evolution de la mortalité périnatale dans une maternité de moyenne importance*, thesis, Tours, 1973).

Chapter Three
WHO PRECEDED LEBOYER?

And yet Leboyer's suggestions are nothing new. They have been expressed by other people, but either they were less vocal or less credible, or the times were not right. Who came before Leboyer?

As early as the 14th century a monk named Bartholomew the Englishman realized how important it was that the newborn baby should be given a warm and muted darkness like that inside the maternal womb: 'It must be put in a dark place to sleep and better to confine its sight.' When discussing birth without violence and the subdued lighting favored by Leboyer, allusions are sometimes made to the practices of the Easter Islanders who expose their newborn babies to daylight only over a period of time, with the result that their night vision is supposed to be exceptionally good.

The true precursor of Leboyer in the 20th century is Maria Montessori. In around 1930 she wrote of the newborn child, 'He arrives in the adult world with delicate eyes which have never seen daylight and ears which have never known noise. His body, hitherto unbruised, is now exposed to rough contact with the soulless hands of an adult who disregards that delicacy which should be respected . . . So, we do not understand him. For us he is not a man. When he arrives in our world we do not know how to receive him; and yet the world we have created will be his, it is he who must continue it and take it further along the road to progress than we have done' (*L'Enfant*, 1975).

Writing in the French journal *Bionaturisme* in 1954, R. Destreit commented on birth and trauma:

All the cares lavished on the baby from the moment it appears only serve to tilt it towards departure. When the baby arrives there is a shock waiting for it. More, a series of shocks.

After several months in the calm, silence, dark and comfortable softness of the mother's womb, the baby is suddenly and abruptly made aware of noise and light in an ambient temperature around 15-20 degrees lower than that it has known during those nine months. As if this rush of shocks was not enough, it is then exposed to the particularly brutal treatment of an early cutting of the umbilical cord.

How could the newborn child be impervious to this sudden transition from dark to light, from silence to noise, from warmth to relative cold . . .?

Perhaps all babies would see from birth if they were habituated to light in a more gradual manner. We do not know how many cases of deafness may result from damage to the hearing organs by over-sudden noise.

Instead of thinking about all these vital precautions, we concentrate on microbes. Instead of trying to protect and develop all the marvellous natural immunities, we kill all the microbes without wondering what may happen to their corpses as the blood carries them away. As soon as the baby is born, it becomes a field of battle between nature and the laboratory. It is cleaned with disinfectant solutions, powdered with sinister antiseptic talc. It has a terrible caustic, nitrate of silver put into its eyes which will weaken its sight and its defences (perhaps for life) by destroying a number of tiny beneficent organisms.

Then there are the barbaric modern methods of inducing labor when the operator decides the time is right. It is no longer we who suit ourselves to the child's needs, but the child who adapts to ours. And by delaying its first cry and destroying nerve cells, all these practices may inflict such irreparable havoc that the effects will last throughout the baby's life.

For the moment we will go no further, hoping perhaps presumptuously that we have drawn the reader's attention to one aspect of the human problem which men of science believe they have solved.

Towards the end of his life Wilhelm Reich sought the reasons for this massacre of the innocents, this apparently universal hatred of the child. He addressed himself to the Little Man or *homo normalis* i.e. the 'miserable and small, stinking, impotent, rigid, lifeless and empty' man: 'But when I think of your newborn children, of how you torture them in order to make them into 'normal' human beings after your image, then I am tempted to come close to you again, in order to prevent your crime.' Reich knew that the Little Man has lost the ability to love. 'You can only ladle in and only take, and cannot create and cannot give, because your basic bodily attitude is that of holding back and of spite; because panic strikes you when the primordial movement of love and giving stirs in you. That is why you are afraid of giving. For the same reason you keep running away from the truth, Little Man: it might release the love reflex in you' (*Listen, Little Man,* 1948). Reich's ideas open the way to interesting lines of research. His chief thesis and the basis of 'bio-energy' is the theory that the conflict between desire and its repression, masked by the subject's history and social conditions, leaves its mark on the body. The working hypotheses recently developed by Goodfield are obviously inspired by Reich. Goodfield suggests that memory is not confined to the brain, but that every cell in the body retains a memory of the pleasure and pain it once felt, whether in early infancy, at birth or in the womb. In order to elicit these memories from the cell Goodfield uses a combination of hypnosis and thermography to show up heat variations on the surface of the body.

In his book *The Death of the Family* (Penguin 1971) David Cooper questions the process of education. It is he who offers a much wider view of preparation for birth.

> We are in fact dealing here with a critical phase of education, but education in ambivalent sense. It is education for the emerging person interacting with education for the mother and the doctor and the midwife. Education for the adults means most immediately being open to the experience of the infant in the sense of allowing experiential resonances to reach down to their own birth experiences which I believe are more *taught out* of them by a highly conscious mis-educational process than repressed in the familiar psychoanalytic sense.

David Cooper wonders how we can have forgotten 'coming into the world of garish clinical light into dutiful undelighted hands, the clanging of chromium instruments.'

Michel Bataille strikes a humorous note in his novel *Le Soleil Secret.*

> You suffocate, you do not wish to leave, you are right, no use, you are half strangled, your sides squeezed in a

vice, your chest half flattened ... Finally your head emerges. Ouch. You are cold, in pain, you would like to die ... Then, by way of a welcome, a gesture of friendship, to show you the ways of this planet where you haven't asked to come, do you know what the doctor does? He picks you up by your feet, holding both ankles in one hand, and with the other he smacks you a couple of times ... or spanks you on the buttocks, both methods have their own champions. To help you breathe ... would you believe? If, after that, you haven't understood, you must be completely stupid.

Among the less obvious precursors of Leboyer we might also number Joan Grant, a medium who believes she has relived all her past lives from Antiquity to the present day, and her husband Denys Kelsey, a psychiatrist who used hypnosis to make his patients relive their past lives and discovered that psychoses and neuroses come from unconscious memories of previous existences.

Their book *Many Lifetimes* (Gollancz, 1968) includes the following passage:

From infancy most of us are deprived of the identification provided by skin-to-skin contact – although this is sometimes prescribed for delicate babies under the chilling heading of T.L.C., 'Tender Loving Care'. Very few children have the natural solace of being caressed in mutual nakedness, even by their parents: so it is not in the least surprising that they grow up with such a pressure of unsatisfied longing ...

Of birth itself they write:

Voices should be hushed and the clatter of instruments on stone floors, the banging of doors and so forth should be avoided. It would be a kindly gesture to reduce the lighting as the baby's head is on the point of emerging ... The baby should be placed naked against the naked chest of the mother. A screen arranged across the waist of the mother would then shield the baby when the lights are restored to full power so that the technical aspects of the delivery can be completed. The baby can be given its first bath at leisure, but then should be returned to naked contact with the mother. Skin-to-skin contact is such a vital means of transmitting a feeling of security to a baby that far more use should be made of it, especially during feeding. I believe it is also important that the baby should always be within sounds of a friendly adult. The custom which prevails in some maternity establishments of allowing the babies to howl their heads off unattended in a separate nursery has nothing to recommend it.

To return to the more scholarly and serious, it is worth mentioning Otto Rank's work *The Trauma of Birth* (1929). In fact, Rank is in no sense a true precursor of Leboyer who deplored anything which might wilfully produce additional postnatal traumas. Even so, the *Trauma of Birth* is important for its historical role within the psychoanalytic movement because it is the first work to have stressed the relationship with the mother. It should be regarded as one aspect of the search for the biological origins of neuroses.

Rank's dogma is based on one observation in particular: that during the final phase of analysis, the cure often emerges from the unconscious in the symbolic form of birth. The patient's desire to be cured is expressed in the fantasy of second birth from which s/he then emerges to regard himself or herself as the spiritual child of the analyst. The ultimate effect of analysis is to free the patient from the obsession with the trauma of birth. Rank attributes a fundamental importance to birth trauma, its repression and reappearance in neurotic reproduction, symbolic adaptation, moral reactions, aesthetic idealization and philosophical speculation. As Rank sees it, any human creative activity of some social value, including humanization itself, must be regarded as the product of a specific reaction to the trauma of birth. These arguments may be open to question since their author is an artist rather than a scientist, but they do at least deal with the little-known reality surrounding birth. In a study of the predisposition to anxiety, Phyllis Greenacre takes up the question of the relationship between birth and anxiety and recalls that Freud had himself criticized Rank's theories with which he disagreed (*Trauma, Growth and Personality*, 1953).

More recently, through the discovery of 'primal pain', Janov has urged us to reconsider the role of the pain associated with birth. In primal therapy the curative agent is pain. Its expression is a deep, involuntary scream which resembles a death rattle. The scream is produced when the patient's defences have been abruptly shattered and s/he suddenly finds herself or himself naked before suffering, entirely exposed to the truth. Some patients have been able to relive what appeared to be their birth at the first session (an experience also open to takers of LSD, those who practice bio-energy and followers of traditional eastern methods). Others had primals which went further and further back into their past (*The Primal Scream*, 1970). It is still difficult to evaluate the full implications of primal therapy.

Of all Leboyer's precursors, however, Bernard This in

his book *Naître* (1972) has been the only writer to lay such stress on birth, an experience common to us all, and to title his work 'naître', a verb in the active voice which means 'to be born'. This valuable and historic book centres attention not on the mother but on the baby which 'is not a manufactured object produced by the mother like a cake out of the oven. It is growing, developing and, at the moment of birth, it has its own statement to make even as it lies, mouth open, unwrapped, the first cry over, simply breathing. If delivery is the business of the mother who brings it out of her body and offers it to the father, then birth is the business of the baby.' The words of Bernard This stand as the ultimate condemnation of our massacre of the innocents:

We can always talk about loving our neighbor, organize conferences and congresses, discuss respect for the human individual until we're blue in the face, denounce a world of concentration camps, condemn slavery, colonialism, torture, the exploitation of man by man; it all helps to salve our consciences. But what are we doing in our families, in our nurseries, or in our hospitals? Who is the real Herod?

Chapter Four
FEELING AND REASON

It was then that Leboyer arrived.

What conscious and unconscious reasons led us first to read, then to accept and finally to accord so much importance to a short book apparently written for the general reader? Without doubt, we were ready for it in some ways. But it was women who actually enabled us to understand Leboyer so quickly. Obviously there are some men who have responded sympathetically to his book, possibly those who can relate to others without necessarily taking up the defensive posture usually regarded as manly. But it seemed significant that such a large number of women, and particularly pregnant women, should have immediately adopted such a positive attitude to Leboyer's work. We were reminded of the power of knowledge by instinctive emotional fusion described by Max Scheler in his book *The Nature of Sympathy* (1970). According to Scheler the average adult man living in an advanced civilization has to a large extent lost that mode of knowledge which is found in animals, children, dreamers, some neurotics, subjects under hypnosis and in primitive man. Some women, on the other hand, still have a power of knowledge based on maternal instinct which exists in man, and particularly civilized man, only in a quite rudimentary state. This power of emotional fusion, although based in actual or potential motherhood, can extend into many areas.

Alerted by women, then, we listened to Leboyer who speaks to us not as a scientist addressing the intellect but as a man appealing to our feelings. And having listened we began to imitate. All our staff, which consists mainly of women, were quick to understand the importance of the changes taking place. Alongside our emotional responses we were also developing reasoned arguments to support them, or perhaps to justify them *a posteriori*.

Our reasoned arguments were based on one key notion: that the first hours and days following birth have a determining and irreversible influence on the future. And this notion has been the focus for a variety of apparently very disparate disciplines.

Nutritionists and dieticians, for example, tell us that the adipocytes or fatty cells in the newborn baby do not keep their ability to increase mass by multiplication for very long. Obesity is therefore determined to a certain extent during the first days of life.

Endocrinology is continually producing new evidence to show how the hypothalamo-hypophysial system of the newborn baby, which probably plays a vital role in triggering off labor, is regulated and adjusted according to the first environmental experiences. All this evidence suggests that the behavioral characteristics of the individual will depend to a large extent on the adjustments which then take place. It is during this period of neo-natal regulation that the primitive reptilian brain, the hypothalamus, adopts a mode of activity which is either feminine, discontinuous and cyclic if the degree of male hormonal impregnation is low, or masculine and continuous if the degree of male hormonal impregnation is high. To put it in a more general way, endocrinology shows that certain anomalies in adult behavior can be induced or programmed from birth. At the moment endocrinologists are also examining the symbiosis which persists between mother and child after birth. Unexpected variations in the maternal curve of adrenal hormone elimination, for example, often lead to an exactly corresponding change in the infant curve. The school of Besancon has shown that when the mother was 'available' with a high appeasement/aggression coefficient, synchronization was virtually complete.

Immunologists have shown that caressing promotes the manufacture of antibodies in the newborn rat, and the importance of the immune system in infectious disease, rheumatology, oncology and allergology is now totally accepted.

Neurophysiologists show how important the first hours and days outside the uterus are by singling out the human baby as a special case because its prolonged neural immaturity makes it more deeply susceptible to the modelling and structuring influences of the environment. As soon as the baby is born, interaction structures the development of its intelligence and emotional life. The final maturing process of the baby's brain takes place in a social environment. Although the newborn human has a definitive number of grey cells at birth (around 14,000 million, four times more than a chimpanzee), the pathways between cells are by no means laid down and almost all the linkage remains to be established. This extraordinary network of fibres, which is gradually covered with a sheath of myelin, begins to form at around the seventh month of intra-uterine life and is completed around the age of 14 years. Neurophysiologists have recognized the effects of starting up brain activity too early through environmental stimuli and the serious conse-quences of emotional and sensory deprivation on later epigenetic development. Significantly, physiologists like Hans Seyle believe that the response to stress can be engendered not only by an excess but also by a lack of external demands, both physical and psychical.

In his study of the development of auditory function, A. A. Tomatis, a hearing specialist, has also revealed the importance of birth in conditioning future life. ('Comment l'enfant nait aux sons', in the journal *Son*, November 1972). In the uterus, the outer, middle and inner ears are adapted to the same frequencies which are roughly those of water, i.e. mostly over 8000 hertz. At birth the baby enters a new sonic environment: the outer and middle ears will have to adjust to the impedances of the air while the inner ear remains in a liquid medium. In fact, the first hours and days following birth are a period of transition during which the middle ear, and in particular the eustachian tube, still contain amniotic fluid, so that to start with, the middle and inner ears remain attuned to the same frequencies as before. After the second day the eustachian tube is emptied of liquid, the baby loses its perception of high-pitched sounds and can hardly hear at all. Then gradually around an axis between 300 and 800 hertz the ear drum opens to the world of sound, and the infant rediscovers its mother's voice, re-experiencing an auditory perception it has known during its fetal life. Obviously the mother's voice sounds very different, but the baby can recognize its inflections and rhythms. Tomatis believes this vocal 'food' to be as necessary a part of our human structuring as the milk we drink. There is an 'ideal sonic progression' which affects not only how we hear but also how we speak and read.

Walter Howard, a musicologist who has attended many births and observed many newborn babies, confirms that the first auditory impressions are the most important.

Ethnology allows us to establish a relationship between

the attitude of a given society towards children and the degree of violence observed in adults. In an article on this subject entitled 'Body Pleasure and the Origins of Violence' (*Bulletin of Atomic Scientists*, November 1975) James Prescott compared the behavior of 49 primitive societies. His study leads inevitably to the conclusion that our only hope of preventing violence lies in greater awareness of the early determining significance of physical pleasure in general and the pleasures of touch, contact and body movement in particular.

By the very nature of its subject matter psychoanalysis bases its doctrines on the important effects of early infancy. Since Freud, many people have accepted the idea that the conscious mind develops from the unconscious and Freud himself compared the analyst's work of reconstruction with that of the archaeologist. It was Freud also who paved the way for analytical observation of babies with the case of Little Hans and who encouraged the pursuit of similar studies in the hope of deriving therapeutic and educative applications from them. The many people who have worked in this field have confirmed Freud's discoveries and attached increasing significance to the first hours and days of life. Melanie Klein has shown the fundamental importance of the baby's first object relation, the relation to the mother's breast and to the mother, and has enabled us to see that the complexity of the mature personality can only be comprehended from the psyche of the newborn infant and its development throughout life. As she sees it, the different stages in libidinal development can be envisaged less in serial terms than in terms of mutual interpenetration. She attributes a higher degree of ego organization to the infant than does Freud and suggests that from the moment of birth the child can be exposed to very real anxieties and yet capable of confronting them through already well-developed defense mechanisms. The Oedipus complex then marks the culmination of a long process which begins during the first moments of libidinal organization at birth. By constructing his own analyses and his own vocabulary, Winnicott has made a useful contribution to our understanding of the mother-child relation, particularly as regards the vital importance of its initial phase. During the first hours and days the mother's task is to create the illusion that her breast is part of the infant, which requires almost one hundred per cent adaptation on her part to start with. She must then gradually disillusion the infant, but success here will be correlated to the opportunities for illusion she has already created.

In other words, the infant acquires a certain ability and a certain need to love from birth, and it is from this ability that the breast is then created and recreated. A good mother, therefore, is a person who will adapt herself entirely to the needs of the child at the beginning. Subsequently, as the child becomes able to permit less adaptation and to tolerate the effects of frustration, the mother needs adjust less. (In psychoanalytic terms, breast can be taken to mean mothering behavior in general. Bottle feeding need not necessarily therefore preclude good mothering.) This theory of the illusion-disillusion process enables us to understand the consequences of insufficient mothering at the critical early stage which may be difficult to reverse later on. In France, Françoise Dolto has emphasized the importance of the newborn's first breaths and singled out the respiratory stage. During its first hours the newborn baby is submerged under a wave of sensory information, basically olfactory and tactile which is the child's way of getting to know the world. Breast feeding also brings the baby a smell of its mother and a sense of tactile well-being.

Although psychoanalysis was almost the only discipline to concern itself with early infancy until the middle of this century, the rapid development of ethology which uses observation of animals, sometimes in experimental conditions, has changed the picture. Obviously we should avoid the unthinking use of ethological discoveries lest we fall into what might be called the zoomorphic trap. There can only be analogies between animal models and human behavior, not equations. The difference between animals and humans is that, once the learning period is over, the animal code of behavior is fixed according to a kind of ritual peculiar to its particular group. The human code is constantly evolving, since language enables us to conceptualize and develop. One of the most striking characteristics of our time is the conception of language as the 'key' to humankind and to social history. Using their own language and their own methods of research, the ethologists emphasize the extent to which initial environmental experiences determine all subsequent behavior by leaving their mark on a sensitive period in the maturation of the nervous system, the period of 'imprintability'. Thus a jackdaw reared by a human being during its period of imprintability (13-16 hours after hatching) will live normally with other jackdaws; but in the mating season its sexual feelings will be directed solely towards humans and not to partners of its own species. By re-establishing the long-neglected link between animal infancy and human infancy, the ethologists have contributed to our understanding of the origins of emotion. Psychologists who use ethological concepts see attachment not as the result of a learning process, of reinforcement, but as a primary need: in the newborn baby the need for contact, the search for closeness to the mother, is greater than hunger. In a more general way, ethologists observing birds, mammals and, in particular, primates, have noted forms of behavior which have nothing to do with physiological needs but are social in function. A number of experiments in mother-child separation in animals has confirmed that, as in the case of human babies, loss of the mother gives rise to potentially irreversible problems. Marshall Klaus has shown that at the beginning of life there is a very sensitive period when separation is particularly damaging. When mother goats and sheep are separated from their young for no more than a few hours immediately after birth, their subsequent ability to mother is unmistakably impaired. Marshall Klaus has also studied the long term effects of early separation in humans by identifying and comparing three groups of mothers of premature babies: those who were allowed into the special care baby unit on the fifth day after birth, those who were not allowed in until the twentieth day and those allowed in on the fortieth day. There was also a control group of mothers who did not go into the unit at all but whose babies were cuddled every day by a nurse. Needless to say, there were marked differences between the three groups. Ethology, too, shows the first hours after birth to have a determinant and irreversible influence on the future of the individual.

If the first hours have such a profound influence on the future of the individual, what can we say about the future of the species?

Here, too, experimental psychology or ethology may provide a better answer than clinical observation by examining the acquisition and inter-generational transmission of the capacity to mother. This, the most archaic form of the ability to love, the most archaic form of all human relations, is acquired very early in infancy. It is from their own birth that females learn to mother. Mothering behavior is passed down from mother to daughter in a congenital rather than a chromosomatic way. When mothering behavior is disturbed, the effects are ineradicable and the traumas are also passed down from mother to daughter.

The real significance of the ethologist Harlow's work in 'The nature of Love' (*American Psychologist, 13,* 1958) has been recognized by R. Zazzo who described 1958 as a year memorable for the union of infant psychology with ethology. For in that same year, Bowlby, the psychoanalyst known for his work on infant disturbance due to lack of maternal care, published an article which went beyond the generally accepted theses on the subject ('The Nature of the Child's Tie to his Mother', *International Journal of Psycho-Analysis, 39,* 1958). Harlow specialized in the study of the young rhesus monkey. His experiments with artificial mothers are among the most significant. Small monkeys were reared by artificial mothers, some made out of wire netting, others covered in fur, from which the young were able to get bottled milk round the clock. These mothers were endlessly patient, never angry, immobile, soundless, constantly emitting the same smell, never cradling their young. By this means Harlow was able to study the importance of nestling and the respective importance of maternal affection and attachment to peers. After three months of isolation, some monkeys survived and could be 'recuperated' by group psychotherapy, i.e. by contact with young monkeys of their own age. Most importantly, some of the monkeys reared in this way, experimentally traumatized and then recuperated, could become mothers in their turn. Some did refuse all sexual contact, others became pregnant only to abort, but several were able to continue their pregnancies to term. It was thus possible to observe the behavior of mothers traumatized in infancy by lack of their own mothers. Some were indifferent and passive like the artificial mothers; others were aggressive, crushing their young's head on the ground, unable to tolerate juvenile cries and games; others were able to bear a second baby and they behaved either normally or hyperprotectively.

Confirmation of the results recorded in these experiments comes in various other works. Kaufman and Rosenblum, for example, have studied mother-child separation in the cynopithecus and pig-tailed macaque. In any discussion of the future of humanity, however, we must beware of making overhasty extrapolations from animal to human behavior since humans benefit from the tool of language which helps to develop and convey cultural phenomena.

We have now reached the culmination of those rational arguments which have served as complement to and justification for the feelings Leboyer inspired in us.

We start from various presuppositions: first, that Freud was right in prescribing that the human masses 'join together libidinally'; second, that love is the major if not the only factor in civilization since it influences the transition from egoism to altrusim; and third, that hatred and rivalry can only be moderated by new political and economic structures inspired by the spirit of love. It then follows that a knowledge of the way the ability to love and to mother is passed on from one generation to the next is of fundamental importance. Do obstetricians realize the probable extent of their responsibility for this transmission of the ability to love?

Psychosomatic medicine, or rather the psychosomatic approach to certain illnesses, also helps us to perceive the determining influence of the first parent-child relation. As a surgeon I have been brought face to face with the basic concepts of psychosomatic medicine, particularly in connection with duodenal ulcer. In fact, there are several schools of thought which recognize the part played by the nervous system in the pathogenesis of the duodenal ulcer. Although not entirely discredited, Pavlov's cortico-visceral doctrine, Seyle's adaptation syndrome and the theory of personality profiles have been eclipsed and superseded by psychoanalytically inspired ideas and in particular by the compelling theories of Alexander (*Psychosomatic Medicine,* New York, 1950). Alexander has shown that it is not the personality type but the kind of conflictual situation which is decisive. What makes his theory both original and interesting is the emphasis he places on the oral phase in libidinal development. During the first phase, the newborn child feels pleasure when it is fed, and during this stage of dependence on its mother, being fed and being loved are indistinguishable. Later, the desire to remain in a state of infantile dependence, to be loved and cherished, may come into conflict with the adult self, its sense of pride and its desire for independence. Certain patients seek to avoid this conflict and to take refuge in a situation of dependence by regressing. In most cases, however, it is impossible to return to the symbolic protection and nourishment of the mother. It would seem that the crucial factor in the pathogenesis of the ulcer is the frustration of desires for dependence, affection and support. Because of the infantile love-food equation, this desire for dependence becomes a desire to be fed which acts constantly on the stomach through the neuro-vegetative vagus nerve disturbing the regular gastroduodenal functions and secretion of gastric juices.

Alexander's theories have sometimes been criticized in psychoanalytic circles, by Grinker for example. Some people, such as Ziwar and Marty, have amended or developed his ideas. Nevertheless, they still serve as a reference. In fact, the most detailed work on the connections between psychological disorders and gastroduodenal ulcers has been done by Angel Garma who bases his work on Kleinian teaching (*La Psychanalyse et les ulcères gastro-duodénaux*, 1957). Discussing a concrete case treated by psychoanalysis for five sessions a week over three years, Garma reveals some of the unconscious processes which give rise to the ulcer and details his theory of the 'internalized bad mother' aggravating the digestive system and manifesting in the patient an instinctual oral and digestive regression. The image of the mother is like a form of toxic food. Garma appositely quotes the verses of Lawson:

> I cannot eat but little meat
> My stomach is no good.
> The pain I get and oft repeat
> Depends upon my mood.
> I've always had a strong conceit.
> I cannot tolerate defeat.
> It all dates back to mother's teat
> And acids all my food.

Whatever the variations in details between these different interpretations, there is no question but that the initial phase of the mother-child relation plays a significant part in the pathogenesis of the ulcer; a fact which obstetricians would do well to consider.

Certain aspects of ulcerous disease are still virtually unexplored, particularly the longterm future of the duodenal ulcer which is treated in conservative fashion following perforation in the peritoneum, or rather the future of the patient after the drama of perforation. At all stages of technical development in surgery from 1925 to 1975, certain surgeons have attested to cures in a majority of ulcer patients when accidental perforation was treated by suture alone. However, there have always been a large number of surgeons who were so convinced that secondary radical surgery would be necessary during the months following perforation that they have performed such surgery in the first place, either in the form of gas-trectomy, or as mostly happens now, gastrectomy or vagotomy.

Working in the surgical department of a small provincial hospital from 1963 to 1968, I personally treated 22 perforated duodenal ulcers by suture. All these cases were then followed up so that we could measure the longterm effects. Only one underwent secondary surgery. In most large teaching hospitals, however, surgeons increasingly opt for radical surgery at the outset. It is tempting to see a connection between the variety of psy-chological atmospheres which may surround patients hospitalized for perforated ulcers and the extraordinary divergency of observations made by surgeons concerned with the future of patients after perforation.

Might the drama of perforation (perhaps a re-birth?) call for 'good mothering' above all else? Can we regard this abdominal drama as a period of crisis when the patient is more responsive, more susceptible to emotional alteration? It is possible that the anonymous surgical departments in large hospital emergency wards would find it more difficult than we do to create a therapeutic atmosphere for ulcer patients during an important stage in their psychological life.

We have taken the bulbous duodenal ulcer as typical of somatoneuroses because it is a condition which is frequently encountered by surgeons and because its psychic co-determination has been especially thoroughly examined.

In fact, it has been found that characteristic disturbances in the mother-child relation lie behind all somatoneuroses and it would be equally justifiable in this context to mention the works of Alexander, Schellac, Murray and Mahoney on the subject of ulcero-haemorrhagic colitis. Indeed the whole field of psychosomatic medicine needs to be re-examined to take account of the circumstances of birth.

Once the most prevalent conditions of birth have been condemned and a great deal more thought has been given to the initial phase of the mother-child relation, it will surely be possible to develop more fruitful theories about alcohol and drug addiction. The present tendency of the medical establishment to treat addiction as a crime or a disease must cease. Can we really continue to treat the addict as a victim of vicious tendencies or alimentary and metabolic disease? Over fifty years ago there were some people who had glimpsed the truth. Writing about the sufferings of a baby fed by a wet-nurse, Groddeck said, 'He began to drink, a fate which often befalls those who have been forced to do without affection during the first weeks of their life'. In fact it was Sandor Rado who introduced the idea of specifity in addiction as early as 1923. He was the first to try to analyze the mechanism of repeated drug use by asking what kind of subject might be led to drug addiction. His study of pharmacothymia directed him towards the problem of oral eroticism and the discovery that the stimulation process in oral eroticism cannot be confined to the area of the mouth as a somatic source. From this developed the fundamental notion of the alimentary orgasm, the nucleus central to those genital fantasies which are part of infantile sexual theory. Rado believed that the psychic manifestations of oral eroticism also exist in cases of habituation to drugs when they are not orally administered.

All the evidence now suggests that the factors which predispose people to addiction will be found during the earliest stages of libidinal development. While drug addiction in general is one of the major concerns of the world today, as more research is conducted into the pathology of infants born to drug-taking mothers, the subject also becomes especially interesting to obstetricians. It is worth emphasizing how large a number of affected babies there are in technologically advanced countries because the problem affects both present and future generations. American researches have shown that pregnant women take an average of four or five different medicaments during their pregnancy of which 80% are not prescribed by a doctor. Obstetricians have encountered the 'impregnation syndrome' in newborn babies of mothers using depressants of the central nervous sytem or morphine derivatives. These babies exhibit insufficient respiratory movement, hypotonocity, hyporeflexes, a tendency to hypothermia which may make resuscitation in the delivery room additionally complicated. Moreover, such babies are often hypotrophic and risk developing hypoglycemia. Paediatricians are familiar with the privation or weaning syndrome which always appears after a period of latency and is characterized by symptoms of cerebral irritation and digestive troubles which lead to the danger of fatality. Needless to say, the survivors are often victims of emotional or psychomotor disturbances. Although the study of addiction is concerned chiefly with alcoholism, drug abuse and the use of various kinds of depressants, there are other comparable addictions which are part of people's everyday lives. In this connection we would single out tobacco addiction, a subject which has given rise to more theoretical work of late, although it is certain that the oral phase of libidinal organization also needs to be investigated.

It is clear that all manifestations of psychosomatic disturbance should be examined in the light of birthing conditions. If we are to follow Leboyer in introducing Eros into the delivery room, we must inevitably consider the sexual activity of the adult and that vast branch of medicine which now deals with the classification of sexual dysfunctions in women (such as frigidity and vaginism) and in men (impotence, premature ejaculation).

In this connection it is worth recalling the important work done by H. and M. Harlow, since their studies indicate where we should be looking for prophylaxis in the field of sexual function pathology. Harlow's monkeys, reared by artificial mothers, develop sexual troubles as adults. The jackdaw fed by a human 13-16 hours after hatching will only be able to feel adult sexual emotions for a human. A psychoanalytic interpretation will reach the same conclusion. Psychoanalysts following Abraham confirm that premature ejaculation in particular represents a fixation on urethral eroticism. This libidinal fixation is usually reinforced by enuresis and masturbation, and leads to an unconscious identification of sperm with urine which provokes the desire for immediate elimination as soon as any pressure is felt. This means that premature ejaculation occurs because the active, aggressive component of the sexual drive has not been integrated into the primary tendency for passive elimination, and without this integration the penis will not be able to function as a primarily genital organ. To put it in a more general way, impotence, premature ejaculation and all sexual dysfunctions have their origin in difficult relations with the mother. Indeed, at the International Congress of Medical Sexology held in Paris in July 1974, Mme Dreyfus-Moreau summed up her ideas about female responsibility for male impotence in one sentence: 'Give us good mothers and we will have no more impotent husbands.' This statement raises another problem concerning the aims and effectiveness of sex education which is usually received at a very late and developed stage of people's sexual lives. Obviously there is room for the kind of teaching which seeks to inspire responsibility rather than to instruct, which enables adolescents to ask questions and to talk, but we should be aware of its limitations. There is another form of sex education that is worth considering. Indeed it may well be the only real sexual education inasmuch as learning is a product of experience rather than information. We refer here to education during pregnancy, i.e. during a period of crisis when people are open to emotional alteration. At this time it may be possible to reappraise the past, to relive stages of women's lives which were not originally experienced in a satisfactory way.

Mme Dreyfus-Moreau's words also reveal the limitations and problems of all sexual therapy, whether it be the educative technique of Masters and Johnson who overlook the etiology of dysfunction to concentrate on the sexual function itself, or the so-called 'California technique' which ignores both individual existential problems and the interplay of the couple. Anyone who believes that humans start learning about love at birth and that the initial stages of libidinal organization are the basis for the later emotional and sexual life of the adult will find all forms of sexual therapy, however effective in part, very much a last resort. Primal therapy may possibly offer an interesting approach to such problems.

The fact remains that in the field of sexual dysfunction the emphasis should be on prophylaxis, and the road to effective prophylaxis also leads to a consideration of the conditions of birth most often practiced today in industrial societies.

Chapter Five
LOVE AND CIVILIZATION

It is impossible to evaluate the true importance of Leboyer and his precursors without considering the extent to which love is seen as an influence in the process of civilization.

Scientists and doctors tend to overlook or discreetly avoid the word 'love', although Lorenz used it to describe relations between birds (in particular jackdaws and geese). For Laborit love is only a word used to mask the search for dominance and the proprietorial instinct, to describe the dependence of the nervous sytem on the gratification another creature may bring within our own territory. This interpretation is painfully objective. But since humankind is characterized by its ability to imagine, and since the human faculty of creative imagination also enables people to find gratification in rejecting the painfully objective, it is probably safe to assume that the word 'love' still has a future.

In fact, behavioral specialists usually prefer less emotionally charged words such as 'attachment' or 'bonding'. Some of the most complex works dealing with human nature manage to avoid speaking of love. An important conference devoted to the 'emotional reactions of the pregnant woman' which was held in Monaco in 1973 never used it. Leboyer has brought us a step further forward by changing the code and subverting our language. Like all poets he feels that any change in life will follow a change of language. 'Man cannot be changed unless his instruments of knowledge, or language, are changed.' Love is a familiar word to Leboyer. However, there are any number of ways in which the word can be understood.

Christians have no difficulty in interpreting it. Love in Christ urges everyone to place the reality of the other's self on the same plane as one's own reality. Buddhists regard love as a technique which allows people to rise above the individual self locked inside them and to cross the bounds of their individuality. In other words, love is the point of departure and not the goal. The 20th century has used various means to understand the profound laws of love. Max Scheler emphasized the ability to discover hitherto unrecognized qualities and values in others which can only be found through love. He sees love not as an emotional state but as the cause of an emotional state, an aim, a spiritual act which reveals higher values to us. Sartrian existentialism saw in it only one aspect of communication with others. Spiritual communion is an illusion. In order to exist, such communion must be the coming-together not of two objects but of two free subjects. But love is both giving and possessing, and by possessing, it necessarily regards the other person as an object, alienating his or her freedom. In Sartre's work this pessimistic analysis is linked to a particular concept of the self as unamenable and uneasy, fearing contact or even attention from others as potential encroachment, seeking to enslave others from the first moments of communication for fear of itself being enslaved. As Emmanuel Mounier put it, relations between the self and the other are like two property-owners quarrelling over some possession, not the exchange of a superabundance between two beings. But if the self becomes open and amenable towards the other, neither calculating nor distrustful, if the relationship becomes an exchange and not merely two-handed egoism, giving rather than possessing, then there is love. Neither Sartre nor Mounier take into account the love of self, the origins of narcissism, the significance of auto-eroticism in relation to love of object. The need for self-love has been best expressed by David Cooper who writes of the 'realization that one can never love another person until one can love oneself enough – on every level including the level of proper (i.e. full orgasmic) masturbation – that is, to masturbate at least once with joy. Without a secure enough base in self-love, one inevitably and repetitively acts out the whole mass of implanted guilt in one's relations with others.'

Psychoanalysis directs us towards the real significance of love by exploring its origins. Love in the adult is the transfer of feelings once felt for the mother. If love is defined as the relation of subject to its sources of pleasure, then for the newborn baby the first source of pleasure is the mother who gives it food, warmth and care. Love, therefore, can only be defined through its origins, by evoking the earliest phase of the mother-child relation. Melanie Klein has shown the importance of later identification with parents and thereafter with others. When identification has attained its goal and its effects last into adult life, it becomes possible to enjoy giving others pleasure as if one was receiving pleasure oneself, by putting oneself in their place. It is our ability to identify, to admire the successes of others, which originates in infancy, that enables us to join in productive team work. We can experience pleasure in working with people who may be more talented than ourselves because we identify with them. Once we see that love in the adult can only be determined through its infantile origins and understand how fruitful team work comes about, then love becomes a

very 'modern' concept. Realistic and positivistic construc-
tions of the world have always ignored love. It should,
however, be occupying the highest rung on our scale of
values, since mere necessity, the mere advantages of
collaboration, are not enough to unite the masses. At a
time when humanity is being forced to confront a
common destiny and must for its own sake carry through
a programme of civilization in order to achieve an essential universality in human social structures, love is a
concept of the present. Problems must be solved by adopt-
ing an attitude of love and altruism, not of everlasting
aggressivity. By understanding this we also see the
importance of Paul Leyhausen's work (*Science, Medicine
and Man*, I, 1974). By introducing the notion of bioethics,
seeking the biological origins of altruism, exposing the
vague definitions on which discussions about aggression
are based and showing that aggression only really exists in
the eye of the beholder, Leyhausen offers a compelling
reply to specialists in aggressivity.

If we accept that the chief function of love is the pre-
servation of the species, if we base our definition of love
on its origins in infancy, remembering that the ability to
love is passed down the generations, and if at the same
time we condemn the present daily practice of obstetrics,
then prognoses about the future of our civilization and
possibly of the whole human race can hardly be optimistic.
Leboyer's desperate appeal takes on a whole new dimen-
sion.

Other people have reached similar conclusions along
apparently different routes. Take, for example, the work in
ethnopsychiatry carried out by Georges Dévereux and
François Laplantine (Dévereux, *Essais d'éthnopsychiatrie
générale,* 1970 and Laplantine, 'L'Ethnopsychiatrie' in

Psychothèque 19, 1973). This pioneering multidisciplinary approach attempts to combine the fundamental concepts of psychiatry (normal and pathological) with ethnology (the universal classification of culture). Such a simultaneous view leads to the notion of 'mad societies', cultures which are suffocating themselves into extinction by removing all individuality and socialization from their component members. Analysis of psychotic cultures and their characteristics brings the ethnopsychiatrists to form a harsh 'ethnodiagnosis' of our society which foresees the present western world sinking into schizophrenia. The observations upon which they base their view stand as arguments for their case:

Our emotional inhibition

We find it increasingly difficult to communicate, to form relationships which are not controlled in advance by the laws of manifestly sadist-anal competition and aggressivity. Some of our behavioral traits are ethnologically and psychiatrically aberrant: coldness, reserve, suspicion of passion and attraction to the cerebral. We are less and less able to attain a joy in living and that profound loving pleasure which is necessary to physical health, either because we are denied opportunities for real emotional commitment, because we refuse to take them, or simply because we are tired.

Schizophrenic dissociation

The techno-rational ideal, symbolized by what Mendel calls 'technophrenia', leads to a separation between the impersonal professional life whose only criterion is efficiency and the more emotional life. We make a pathological and unequally weighted distinction between what we think and what we feel, rather than experiencing the differences between the two as a vitalizing and constructive paradox. While most of our contemporaries remain in the grip of unending technological optimism, there are others, admittedly far fewer, who live in the illusion of a future society which will universally reject technology.

The frenetic psychic structure of contemporary humanity
As the world becomes void, our impulsive energies remain unharnessed and frighteningly isolated because we have no cultural references to give us direction, no sense of space, because time has speeded up to such an extent that what was true yesterday is no longer true today. Moreover, there are many people for whom contact with concrete reality has become non-existent.

The sadist-anal regression of contemporary humanity
In the face of anything which affects our real lives and the political future of our society, we exhibit infantilism. The contemporary adult is stuck in the early pre-Oedipal stage of development, incapable of mastering the technological power which controls his fate, attaching significance in a typically regressive fashion to possessions like cars, paper qualifications, promotion and country cottages.

Frustration machines
The powerful and amoral machines of technico-capitalism stimulate an abundance of pseudo-desires which the vast majority of individuals cannot satisfy, thereby increasing the causes of frustration and tension between individuals who have no cultural ideal in common.

Pathological compensation mechanisms
The outlets by which individuals avoid or defer confronta-

tion with their own anxieties are also pathological: alcohol, tobacco and other drugs, image-makers like cinema and television, childish amusements like slot machines and gambling, sadist-anal use of the car and, for the leisure cowards, the narcosis of the package holiday.

Western civilization's psychotic destruction of its own culture

The only objects we now handle are stripped of any symbolic significance. Contemporary communication is purely functional and sterile, while in all previous societies people entered into relations with the world in a manner which was symbolic.

Artistic products

Artistic products are subject to the same laws of self-inflicted cultural perversion, whether it be the popular culture doled out by machines and received by a passive public, or the product intended for a would-be intellectual élite attracted to everything which is not alive.

The loss of our sense of identity

Our society creates categories of individuals who agree to conform to prevailing models. Those people who attempt to affirm their identity by wearing unorthodox clothes are merely indulging in a form of inverted mimicry which shows how far our psycho-emotional life has regressed and grown inconsistent.

The diagnosis to which these observations lead could equally well be formed by any ethnopsychiatrist, whether European, African or Asian, who works through continual reference to the universal categories of culture and deculturation. There is no basic difference between this

view and our own prognosis, based on the usual conditions of birth, which stresses the Freudian description of
civilization as the work of Eros. The present conditions of
birth are only one aspect of the technophrenia which
directs the way our society is evolving. Leboyer's distinction is that he sounds the alarm and suggests a remedy at
a specific and particularly important point in humanity's
present vicious circle. The ethnopsychiatrists can suggest
only that we become more aware and point to various
possible areas of cure.

Ecologists, too, are making pessimistic predictions
about our civilization. What they foresee is worse than
ethnocide, a term which only emphasizes inter-human
relations, for their fears are of eco-cide or eco-suicide,
terms which encompass the destruction of eco-systems, or
even the whole eco-system of earth. On the surface their
argument seems very different: we are in a finished world.
We have only one earth. The present exponential growth
in population and industry cannot last indefinitely. Society
has lost control of its demography, technology and consumption. We must, as a matter of urgency, recognize that
our planet is one entity and construct the foundations of a
planetary economy. Ecologists list the chief threats and
suggest specific remedies, but they are idealists as much as
scientists. By stopping wastage in industrial societies,
demanding a reduction in labor intensity, imposing
automation and reduced production, creating leisure
rather than unemployment, setting up new kinds of
decision-making and distributive authorities and opposing
the dominance of the profit motive, ecological awareness
succeeds in questioning the very structures of our society.
Like us, ecologists continue their struggle for the sake of
future generations. American Indians, whose ecological

awareness is innate and instinctive, pertinently remark that 'the white man eats his children'. As ecological awareness also implies condemnation of the injustices on which our global hierarchy is based, it shows the major incompatibilities of our world for rich countries to co-exist with the poor. Most importantly, it precludes any use of force as a solution, whether for domination or revenge. Ecological awareness leads to socialism, which we define as the recognition of misery and injustice and the will to remedy them by changing existing political conditions so that a society of reconciliation can be established. On a world scale the Master/Slave struggle must end in reconciliation between master and slave; and this will only happen if there is an ability to love. It is among the dominant that we must first work to redevelop this ability. Ecologists, too, recognize that the love factor is an essential part of any realistic and positive view of the world. It would seem that our civilization can only survive if we follow the utopian precepts of Saint Augustine in his commentary on the First Epistle of Saint John:

> You give bread to whoever is hungry; but it would be better that nobody was hungry and that you gave to nobody. You give clothes to the naked; would that all were clothed and there was no such necessity ... For all these services are responses to necessities. If there are no wretched there will be no more acts of compassion. And if there are no acts of compassion will the fire of love then be extinguished? More real is the love which you bear for a happy man to whom you can render no service; this love will be more pure and more honest. For if you render a service to a wretched man, you perhaps desire to raise yourself above him so that he who has caused you to do good is below you. He

finds himself in need; you have shared some of your fortune with him. Because you have rendered him a service you appear in some way greater than he who receives. Desire that he be your equal . . .

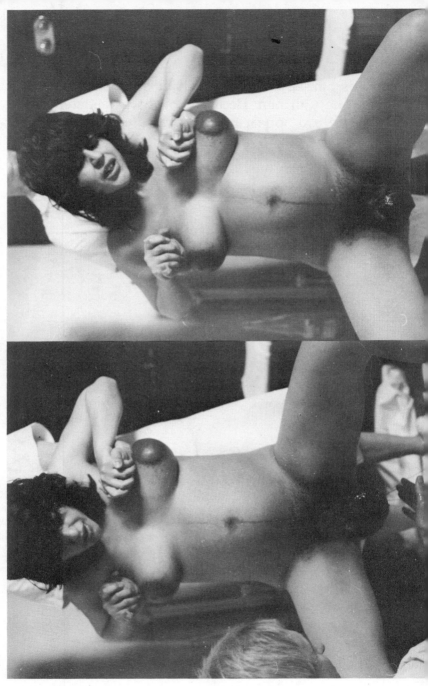

A birth in the squatting position

Part Two
EXPERIENCE

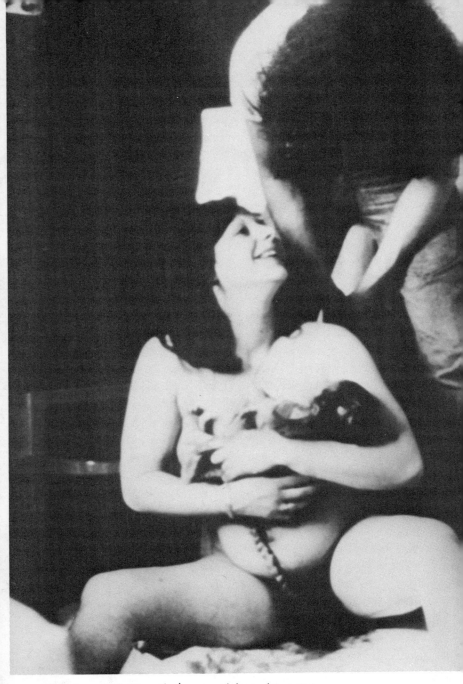

The baby needs first its mother's arms and skin-to-skin contact

Chapter Six
IN THE BEGINNING

Although sympathetic understanding and reasoned argument had some influence, it was Leboyer's book, the film that goes with it and meeting the author that really brought about the change in our maternity unit.

We all realized that Leboyer was not teaching us a method to be followed, but that he was helping us to create a climate, an atmosphere. We all understood that the problems were socio-cultural and not simply medical. We were aware that Leboyer was not asking us to reject the technical, but that he was demanding that we set aside our pride in ourselves as technicians. In early 1974 we focussed our concern on the thirty minutes immediately following birth. We made every effort to avoid any useless gesture which might hamper the development of the parent-child relationship and to end the postnatal trauma which is artificially and gratuitously imposed in most delivery rooms. To do this, we eliminated all unnecessary light sources and observed almost total silence. We insisted that the umbilicus should be left alone while it was still pulsating and that the newborn child should be placed in contact with the mother's belly straight away. We did, however, alter the baby's position here so that it was no longer stretched out on its back (a position condemned by the safety-conscious for any infant likely to suffer temporary breathing difficulty), but laid it on its stomach with arms and legs folded underneath and the head turned to one side, very much like the 'safety position'. To start with, we continued to perform systematic aspiration of the upper breathing passages even when all the evidence suggested that respiration was excellent. We then gave the baby a slow, strong dorsal massage as Leboyer had taught us. Soon we had also adopted the bath, partly perhaps as a gentle transition from the liquid amniotic environment to the aerial environment, partly as a warming process, partly to provide an example of external stimulus as a calming experience and partly as a method of libidinizing the whole skin surface. The perfect adaptation of the newborn to the aquatic environment is well known. Just as a walking reflex can be observed during the early weeks, so, too, will a newborn baby make swimming movements in the water and exhibit a reflex which stops the breathing when the baby is immersed. Fear of water appears to be acquired at a later stage from other people. The early psychomotor development in swimming babies has been emphasized by several scientists.

Before long we gained a better understanding of the newborn. We learned which language the baby would respond to, the importance of touch and skin contact. We saw to what extent the mouth was already differentiated and capable of establishing contact. We observed the archaic reflexes which are given so little room for expression in most delivery rooms, including the rooting reflex which leads the newborn to the mother's breast within minutes of birth. Then we read Leboyer again. We have to read and re-read Leboyer: only he can teach us how to handle the newborn: How should we touch a newborn baby?

Very simply by remembering what it has just left behind. By never forgetting that everything new and unknown may terrify and everything recognizable and familiar is reassurance.

To calm the baby in this strange, incomprehensible world into which it has just emerged, it is necessary – and sufficient – for the hands holding him to speak in the language of the womb.

What does this mean?

That the hands must remember the slowness, the continuous movement of the uterine contraction, the 'peristaltic' wave the child grew to know so well during the final months before birth.

That is another reason why it is necessary to first place the infant on its stomach – so that, by massaging it, we may 'speak' to its back.

What should our hands say? Exactly what the mother and her womb have been saying.

Not the womb as it was during the final labor, not the violent womb that expels and banishes. But the womb of the early, happy days.

The womb that pressed slowly, tenderly. The womb that embraced. The womb that was a source of love.

It was an infinitely sensual amorous relationship that existed between the child and its mother, between the uterus and its prisoner. It is that which must be recreated, to give the baby a kind of soothing echo of what it knew for so long but has now suddenly been taken away, to terrify by its absence.

What is needed is neither a brisk rubbing motion nor a caress, but a deep, slow massage.

Our hands travel over the baby's back one after the other, following each other like waves, one hand still in contact as the other begins. Each maintaining its steady rhythm until its entire journey is concluded.

Without rediscovering this visceral slowness that lovers find instinctively, it is impossible to communicate with the child.

But ... people will say ... 'you are making love to the child!'

Yes, almost.

We have also learned how extremely sensitive newborn babies-are to certain sounds. We have observed Leboyer comforting a newborn baby with gesture and murmur. We have come to know of the tamboura. A discreet tamboura may help to create the right sonic atmosphere for birth. A four-stringed instrument endlessly repeats four notes which can be represented in the tonic sol-fa as *so, doh, doh, so,* the first and last *so* being an octave apart. These four notes form a perfect harmony in which the two outer *sos* unite in the central *dohs.* When the four strings are perfectly tuned, the sound of one makes the three others vibrate as though sympathetically. Listening to this tamboura for just a few minutes can 'induce a sense of inner joy, a fullness, an abundance which must be sung'.

Leboyer revalidates lullabies. Why?

Lullabies are as old as the world, as old as men's suffering and mothers' love.

They rise from others' hearts like the song of the tamboura. What do these lullabies say? The words matter little. Lullabies speak a language which surpasses notes. A language which comes from before Babel. They belong to no religion, no culture, no race.

They speak the language of a land without frontiers which is called the heart of men.

That is why every baby in the world understands them. That is why every woman can sing them.

Nowadays people no longer sing. Machines do it for us. Or pop stars. Women must learn how to sing again. If only to rock their children.

How is a lullaby made? That is a mystery, like the tamboura.

So let the women who have now lost contact with the Source listen to these two lullabies made of four single notes.

Let them come like Savitry Nair into unison with the tamboura and through that harmony into unison with the great harmony.

Let them simply open their mouths and begin to sing. Without useless words. With sounds that rise from their hearts.

Why these bird songs? What have they to do with birth? These bird songs are the songs of our Mother Nature.

Our Mother who supports, shelters and feeds everything that lives without making a sound. From the blade of grass to haughty humanity.

Present day man has lost contact with his mother. He crouches, huddled, in towns.

In those vast cities he can scarcely see the sky, even less the sun. The sound of the wind is lost to him forever. He has forgotten even his mother's voice.

The children now born in these huge prisons are most likely to be testing their ears on the din of traffic.

It isn't possible!

If we have no breeze, no true birds, then here at least are their songs.

So that when they arrive, newborn babies hear something to recall the true land of their birth.

The marvellous serenity Leboyer introduced into the delivery room, which is symbolized by the tamboura, has helped us to recognize and observe the way in which the newborn enjoy sensual pleasure. We have seen the first smile. We have seen how an awakened mouth first discovers the hand, the thumb, or even the mother's breast. We have seen all four limbs gradually and pleasurably stretching and folding as the baby discovers the world. Already it is learning about love at a stage when self-love and object-love are still totally indistinguishable. In the face of such important discoveries, we must surely be moved to silence.

It quickly became clear to us that nothing could be more soothing and comforting for the newborn than its mother's arms. So, after the bath, we dry the baby in a warm towel, form the towel into a hammock which can be rocked and return the child to the comfort of its mother's breast.

Chapter Seven
PREPARATION FOR BIRTH

Such were the immediate, visible changes in our attitude during the first weeks after we had read Leboyer. Before long we had begun to question everything that happened in our unit, to examine its whole justification for existence. Leboyer had been the catalyst for a revolution. It was no longer enough to create a particular atmosphere at the time of birth: there had also to be preparation for this new kind of birth and a continuity between the education and the event.

So, gradually, starting from birth itself, helped perhaps by the dream-like quality of Leboyer's poetry, the maternity unit of our dreams began to grow before our eyes. We have not yet achieved the ideal; perhaps we never will. But we continue to work towards it as we must if the minds of future generations are to radiate a joy in their lives. Preparation for labor has now become a preparation for birth and a learning process for all the adults involved. 'It is not the child who needs preparation. It is we ourselves. If we manifest such blindness, so little understanding in the way we welcome newborn children, can we be surprised that the world is . . . the way it is?'

It is strange that obstetrical prophylaxis should have been confined to so narrow a role over the past twenty years or so. The preparation we follow involves various activities. There are meetings led by a nurse-midwife to which a smallish number of pregnant women come, often with their partners. Weekly groups, at which attendance is strictly voluntary, meet with a psychologist trained in psychoanalysis who, as the mother of three, has experienced different atmospheres for the birth of each of her children. In these groups conversation flows freely between couples expecting a child and couples who have just had a child. It is obvious that the personal experience of a very recent mother will carry more weight with a pregnant woman than any form of formal teaching yet devised. Sometimes these unstructured meetings lead to a sense of community among women expecting to deliver at the same time, who may then support each other. Groups like these offer the best means of profiting from pregnancy as an integrative crisis, a temporary condition which may cause problems for the woman because of her previous experiences.

Frequent access to the place where the child will be born helps to make it familiar. It is important that the maternity unit should not merely be a place where women come for information and examination. That would only make pregnancy seem more like an illness. So our most recent acquisition has been a piano, and the women come here to sing as well.

Of course, an important part of the preparation for the birth is the reading of Leboyer's book by all the staff and the couples involved. We very rarely encounter a pregnant woman who does not immediately connect with the truths in Leboyer's poetry. It is as if the woman's ability to understand were augmented by her condition. Not only are pregnant women able to feel the beauty of the message more clearly than others, they also have a better immediate grasp of its importance. To quote one example: there was a young midwife who read the book for the first time without much interest. She then became pregnant and everything was clear to her. Women learn to transcend taboos, e.g. to touch the baby at birth, by reading or re-reading Leboyer during pregnancy. Annie Lecler's book *Parole de Femme* might have been very different if she had read Leboyer, been prepared for birth and given birth in the right atmosphere. As it is, she wrote, 'And yet it is true, and this is a statement, not a confession, that not once did I think of the child throughout it all. I experienced his birth with him, without thinking of him. It was the midwife who told me that he was healthy and what his gender was; I had not thought to ask. I told myself, the baby born of me is alive; that is all.'

We now see preparation for birth as being the best kind of preparation for labor. In this we agree with Illich that the experience of pain is transformed by industrial civilization into a technical problem to be technically managed. The greater the significance accorded to suffering, the higher the tolerance threshold will become. It is in this sense that preparation for birth transforms the conditions of labor. As Illich points out, apart from the nature and intensity of the stimulus, the experience of pain depends on four factors: culture, anxiety, attention and interpretation. The kind of preparation for birth we practice has an effect on all four of these factors. We have observed that when the woman comes to labor without worrying about her behavior during uterine contractions and how she is controlling them, but concentrating on her baby and how she will welcome it by touch and voice, there is less risk of prolonged or painful labor due to inadequate contractions or anomalies in contraction and dilation. And this applies even where the obstetrical conditions are not particularly favorable, as in cases where the baby's head is presented in the posterior position, for example. Strangely, the use of what we call 'lumbar reflexotherapy' is increasingly rare.

In obstetrics, bilateral lumbar reflexotherapy consists of injecting a very small quantity of sterile water into the thickness of the skin around the kidneys. The injection itself is locally painful but only for a matter of seconds. Lumbar reflexotherapy is effective whenever cervical dilation ceases to progress satisfactorily between 4-6 centimetres and uterine contractions are evident in lumbar pain. Once the back pains have gone, there remains only an ache above the pubic bone, while dilation progresses rapidly. This suggests that the pain itself is an obstacle to dilation. We have used this technique in empirical fashion for a number of years, although some light has now been shed on the possible causes of its effectiveness by Melzac and Wall. By establishing that the gelatinous core which forms part of the posterior horn of the medulla is a complex intregrative system capable not simply of relaying messages to the brain but filtering impulses of pain before transmitting them, they have developed the interesting theory of 'gate control'. This shows an impulse of cutaneous origin might be able to inhibit an impulse of visceral origin. Diminishing use of lumbar reflexotherapy seems to suggest that the conditions which necessitate its use are becoming more rare. And this, in turn, suggests that the two aspects of the obstetrician's role as observer and as technician, are entirely comlementary.

In the delivery room, during the second stage of labor at birth, we have seen a fundamental change in the way mother, father, nurse-midwife and other staff members perceive their respective roles. As a full-time hospital doctor I have no experience of home birth and must therefore work towards bringing the family atmosphere into the maternity unit and ensuring that it is not regarded as just another special department. Through observation we have gained a better understanding of the father's role and of his behavior.

The need for activity on the man's part is something that has been observed throughout the ages, and has even been exploited by some. To quote Joubert: 'Others place the husband's cap or hat on the woman's belly ... But it seems more reasonable to me that the husband himself should cover his wife's belly, since she, by moving however slightly, will gently and enjoyably rock her rump and the husband's seed will make the passage much more slippery than the waters. I know people who act in this way whose wives feel very well and deliver easily.' The usual attitude nowadays to the husband's presence in the labor room is that he is there to help the woman rather than the baby, to be a husband rather than a father. Our view is somewhat different. As we see it, a man who has taken part in preparation for birth is able to be both husband and father, and to play his own special part in controlling the degree of closeness in the mother-child relationship. In some cases the father's role as separator may be more than simply symbolic, and there is no reason why he should not sever the cord. In any case, it is important that birth should not be an entirely two-sided relational phase, isolating mother and child from the rest of the world. The mother needs a point of reference other than her baby. Although it might be supposed that the actual physical presence of the father is not necessary, Tomatis suggests in his theory of the development of language, that the father is probably important as the source of a new voice since the development of social language starts from birth in a desire to communicate with others (*L'Oreille et le Langage*). Anything which impedes the development of the relation with the father may also hamper lateralization (the process by which we become right- or left-handed) and give rise to a fixation at the stage of development where language is created solely for the mother's benefit.

In our unit, anaesthetist and surgical staff have well-defined roles: they are to be available, perfectly equipped, but out of sight. The surgeon should be trained to perform more than simple caesarians. Once the abdominal cavity has been opened there may be all kinds of unexpected problems to deal with. The nurse-midwife is there to act as a calm, discreet and vigilant observer, to offer psychological support to the woman in labor and then to witness the baby's reception by one or both parents. Apart from those cases where caesarian section proves necessary (and ideally this should be decided in advance after considerable deliberation), most obstetrical activity by the staff has no more than historical interest now. The midwife must understand that she has two different but equally important functions, one as a wise and watchful observer ready to raise the alarm, and the other as assistant during the first crucial hours in the mother-child relationship. She must also accept, however, that she will actually be required to 'do' very little, or nothing at all. In this respect our understanding of the role of nurse-midwife or obstetrician reveals a very basic change. In the past human beings have always felt a need for activity during labor. The history of obstetrics is a catalogue of futile and dangerous manoeuvres intended to 'facilitate' labor. This universal need for gestural activity during labor and birth can be seen through a study of language, an analysis of the linguistic unconscious. We have only to look at the language of obstetrics to reveal the mental attitudes underlying this branch of medicine. The idea that the midwife 'delivers' the baby in a transitive sense implies

active intervention. If words are deeds, then we ne
change our language as well as our actions. In our ide
maternity unit (and even that is a misnomer since for us
the unit is first and foremost the place in which the
newborn child begins to develop its personality), we shall
have to develop a new language.

A nurse-midwife who delivers a baby is one who still
thinks it necessary to wear sterile gloves to disengage the
head so that the perineum is protected; whereas in the
vast majority of cases the head will disengage by itself
without any manual intervention and with less discomfort
for the perineum. There may be cases where a little
assistance is required to disengage the shoulders, but
usually the midwife's activities can be confined to placing
the baby on its mother's belly, or helping the father to do
so. The practice of putting on boots, caps, masks and
gloves to perform a delivery is almost laughable when one
considers the numbers of microbes present in the vagino-
vulval and anal areas compared to the negligible
quantity on a clean pair of hands whose contact with the
child's head is in any case very limited. Besides, within a
few seconds of birth the hands holding the baby and the
air around it will no longer be sterile. We work from the
opposing principle and make a point of removing the
paraphernalia of the operating theatre before going to the
delivery room so that we will appear more human.

The word 'obstetrics' and 'obstetrician' are also significant in that they derive from the Latin *obsto* – 'I stand
in front'. We need not dwell on the fact that the word
'obstacle' comes from the same root, but it is worth
remembering where the obstetrician usually stands in relation to the woman and her vulva and that the woman is
usually required to lie on her back, since this is the most

for the use of instruments by the
...re are any number of alternative posi-
...)t. Since it was doctors who imposed
...1 on women several centuries ago, any
doctor's role must now imply a con-
siderat... ...ing positions. *A priori,* the supine position is probably the worst in mechanical terms, since it
makes no use of the force of gravity. The axis of push
makes an angle of 20° with the axis of the upper passage,
so that energy is wasted. Having thought about obstetrical
positions, we have now set up a 'natural' birthing room
quite unlike usual delivery rooms where the woman can
adopt any position she feels like because there is none of
the usual medical furniture. We have also learned to assist
women in seeking alternatives to the conventional lying or
half-sitting. Any position which the woman finds most
comfortable is obviously also the most efficient. However,
while some women choose to squat, to kneel or to sit in a
special chair, others prefer to lie down. Three centuries of
custom will not be eradicated in a few years. Increasingly,
we find that the midwife who has fully grasped her role as
observer, will spontaneously take up a position beside the
woman, from where it is easier to guide and direct her
pushing. The mother, father and midwife will then
experience the birth and discover the child together, side
by side. The fact that we still talk about 'pushing' is due to
our present inability to find new words to describe the
second stage of labor following full dilation of the cervix.
Traditional midwives would tell the woman to 'Push, as if
you were crapping'. This points out the extent to which
this command betrays a confusion between front and back
and regrets the fact that 'expulsion', the technical term,
has connotations of driving out, being rid of. The modern

midwife assisting a well-prepared woman will ask her to breathe in, to block and then to push as she holds her breath. Physiologists rightly point out that these codified commands are not very helpful, and we have been interested to hear of Feijo's use of forced expiration without any real break in respiratory rhythm for women 'sophronized' by sound. As yet we have found no new words to replace 'deliver' and 'obstetrician'. The word natologist sounds too technical. Nevertheless, we must be aware of how inappropriate and potentially dangerous the words we now use may be.

Once the number of professionals present at the birth has been reduced to a minimum (ideally to the nurse-midwife alone), and once their role has been limited to specific activities, birth becomes a family affair again. It is the mother who welcomes the baby and comforts it with touch, gesture and word. There are no technical interruptions of this critical moment in the parent-child relationship. The midwife remains watchful but invisible. 'Whose hands should hold the child? The mother's, of course, provided that these hands know everything we have been saying'. Leboyer had no choice but to receive newborn babies, massage them and speak to them himself. The women who came to him had not been prepared during pregnancy. In our unit, by herself caressing the baby's head, massaging its back, speaking to it and comforting it, not only does the mother stimulate the child's breathing, she also helps the uterus to contract so that the placenta may be expelled. We see increasingly less incidence of artificial delivery. Women with several children who give birth here can remember their feelings after previous deliveries that their babies had been stolen from them. 'After showing me the baby shaded from the light,' wrote one such mother, 'they put it on my belly, and for a moment it was marvellous. But then it was taken away and there is still something empty and shocked about the baby's first half hour which we have not been able to recover. I realize now that I had shut off that moment and that it was mysterious: metallic noises, crying, sounds of water. And then, there I was in a bed with the baby beside me in a cot, all wrapped up with a name bracelet on. There was a distinct separation of mother from child so that from that moment the baby no longer belonged to us. It makes you wonder . . .' This memory of a previous birth raises the problem of transition from the labor room to the room where the mother (or parents) and child stay after birth. Apart from special cases, such as a caesarian, there are no good reasons why mother and baby should be separated at this point. Once any perineal tear or episiotomy has been repaired under local anaesthetic, there are very few mothers who feel unable to walk to their room with their baby in their arms. There should be no abrupt change of hands at this point. If we have managed to keep any expressions of terror and anxiety from the baby's face at birth, why risk inducing them now?

Only with a united team, sharing an identical attitude to birth and an identical way of understanding the baby and the parent-child relationship during the early days can we be sure that an essential continuity is maintained.

MATERNITY UNIT

During your stay in the maternity unit, you will be given every opportunity to look after your baby.

The staff will come between parents and child as little as possible, either in what they do or in advice they may give.

There are no set rules about caring for the newborn baby.

Every baby is a special case.

Nobody knows the real needs of a newborn baby better than its mother.
Be suspicious of spoken or written advice.
Be suspicious of experienced people.
We hope that you will soon feel at home here.

The 'anti-rules', 'anti-information brochure', 'anti-advice' given to couples coming to the unit.

Chapter Eight
A CHANGE?

Our concern to continue into the postpartum period the same atmosphere we have managed to achieve in the birthing room by restricting the number of people present has brought about a change in the whole unit.

Birth Without Violence has made us reconsider the recruitment of staff appointed to work in the unit. Our staff would have to consist exclusively of 'mothers', by which we do not necessarily mean women who have given birth, or even women. In fact, there are considerable problems of the kind that concern anyone whose work involves looking after other people's children. We try to steer a mid-course between two dangerous extremes. There are some people who will feel over-responsible for the child, over-conscious that their experience is greater than the mother's, too sure that they would be the best mother for every newborn baby, sometimes too involved in one particular child. These people will enter into conscious or unconscious rivalry with the mother. Then there are others, possibly more of them, who unconsciously protect themselves from over-involvement and will offer more impersonal, technical, brisk, mechanical and ultimately 'inhuman' care. They are a bad model for the mother to emulate. The behavior of some professional staff who have grown too accustomed to the newborn can only be compared with the conscientious but loveless maternal rearing now known to induce future schizophrenia. In fact, the two extremes we have described here are exaggerations. The nursing staff will always include some people who feel responsible for both mother and child without lapsing into routine and who, however wide their experience, will give every baby its required dose of skin contact, warmth, eye contact and spoken word. Perhaps, however, 'nursing staff' is the wrong definition. Is it really desirable that professionals should come between mother and child? By questioning the role of each member of staff, we have gradually broken down the rigid classification of skills. The psychologist can use a stethoscope, the midwife joins groups for psychoprophylaxis and psychotherapy and maintains her interest in the child until it is several days old; the paediatric nurse can recognize fetal distress during labor; the junior doctor is hoping to specialize in obstetrics and can readily take the midwife's place. By vocation the paediatric nurse and the trainee paediatric doctor concentrate on the newborn child and make a valuable contribution in units usually staffed by people whose present job or past practice has made them primarily interested in the woman. All the men and women in the unit must know how to give artificial respiration to the newborn and how to deal with unexpected respiratory problems. It is easy enough to give lessons on a teaching doll and requires no more effort from the midwife than from the cleaning staff or the doctor. Our staff recruitment is very much part of an overall strategy for institutionalizing birth without violence in a positive sense within a general hospital. To start with, it is enough to advise every member of staff, whatever their duties, to read Leboyer, so that those men and women who are open to his poetry may be identified and helped to progress from an emotional awareness to knowledge of the arguments likely to influence daily practice. Then, as each day passes, an understanding of what birth without violence really means will spread infectiously among their colleagues helped, on occasion, by the couples who come to the unit. Since evolution is inevitable, sooner or later the whole hospital will have shared in the change.

Birth without violence has also given rise to discussions within the team about clothing babies. Obviously we can no longer swaddle a newborn child who has been allowed from birth to explore its entire body in total freedom. We can no longer deprive mother and child of the opportunity for limitless skin contact. Some people have pointed out the more immediate harmful effects of swaddling, such as erythema of the buttocks. But surely Jean-Jacques Rousseau said all that needs to be said: 'When the child breathes as it emerges from its wrappings, do not allow it to be wrapped yet more tightly. No caps, no bindings, no vest but wide-flowing clothes which leave the limbs free and are neither too heavy to hamper movement nor too hot to block the air. Place it in a large, well padded cradle where it can move without harm.'

Thinking about clothes has also led us to consider the shape of the cot (ideally a proper rocking cradle), the bedclothes and the position of the cradle in relation to the mother's bed. Whatever the 'administrative regime' in the hospital, the child should be constantly within hand's reach. It is significant that the demand for private rooms in which mother and child, or parents and child, can be guaranteed total intimacy, is increasing. By keeping mother and child close together we can also help to eliminate strict feeding routines.

When it comes to a choice of feeding methods, we have facts and figures to support our observations. Like many other people, we used to think that the obstetrical staff should encourage breast-feeding and that the best way to do this was by explaining the advantages scientifically and by anticipating and tackling arguments against breast-feeding put forward by reluctant mothers or, as in many cases, by their families and friends. Through birth without violence we have come to see the significance of breast-feeding in a different light. There has been a considerable increase in the number of mothers who breast-feed in our unit, although this is not something that we specifically sought or predicted. The increase has aroused interest among the manufacturers of formula milks. It is worth pointing out that the quantity of breast milk appears greater and the act more satisfying the more emotionally at ease the mother feels. A gentle birth in a delivery room where the emotional climate is right seems naturally to go hand in hand with breast-feeding. This suggests to us that breast-feeding is a symptom of a particular quality in the mother-child relationship. There is no doubt that preparation for breast-feeding begins with the little girl who is fed by her own mother, or who is present when satisfactory breast-feeding occurs. But a woman is most open to influence over her choice of feeding method during the preparation sessions, in the delivery room, and above all, at the moment when her dream becomes a reality. Very few mothers will subsequently refuse to feed a baby who has already found the breast in the labor room.

To quote one young mother:

Oh, the strength of that first sucking! Such spontaneity and strength must be because it is 'natural', or rather necessary. So why don't all newborn babies enjoy it? I would like to know what excuses have been invented for distancing the mother and baby by delaying the first feed for 24 or 36 hours ... I would like to write about that first sucking, but I can't. I would like to be able to translate the power of the emotion I felt into words if only to retain the memory of it ... But that baby's mouth seemed powerful, so strong that it could have been an adult mouth.

Even so, some mothers are still reluctant, badly prepared and ill-informed within hours of birth. It is only then that the basic question has to be asked: will breast-feeding have a good influence on the quality of the mother-child relationship? Obviously the answer is yes when one considers how bottle-feeding imposes a physical distance, reducing both skin contact and the duration of feeding. That physical communication which helps to bring emotional extensions to the mother-child relationship must therefore be encouraged and every effort made to uncover the real reasons why reluctant mothers refuse to feed.

The main argument made against breast-feeding is the need to return to work soon after birth. Here, we can simply explain that six weeks of breast-feeding will give the baby much of the essential benefit inherent in this method and that gradual weaning from breast to bottle two or three weeks before returning to work will cause less serious physiological upsets than bottle-feeding from the beginning.

Another argument, often put forward by a well-meaning family as much as by the mother herself, is the fear of chaps and abcesses. Although it may be inappropriate to insist that any woman who has had problems of this kind with previous babies should try again, first-time mothers can easily be made to see the harmful effects of over-feeding, aggressive marketing by formula manufacturers and rigid routines, associated with bottle-feeding.

Some women may find that malformed nipples are a real difficulty, if not a total obstacle to breast-feeding. They can be taught how to get the whole of the pigmented area into the baby's mouth so that the nipple is in contact with the upper part of the tongue. Sucking will then begin and the resultant stimulation of the pituitary gland will help to trigger off secretion of milk.

The desire to resume taking oral contraceptives need not be an obstacle in itself, though some oral contraceptives themselves are now under serious reconsideration. In many countries breast-feeding remains the most widely used method of regulating birth, but it may be considered insufficiently reliable in industrialized societies. Daily low-dose combination oestrogen and progestogen pills are therefore usually prescribed, although the contraceptive steroids do pass into the mother's milk. It may be better to use other contraceptive methods during the period of breat-feeding.

Caesarians are no prevention to breast-feeding, neither are any of the minor operations a woman may decide to have during the immediate postpartum period, such as sterilization.

In fact, the real reasons for refusing to breast-feed are not usually expressed in any cogent form. The breast as an erotic object has taken over from the breast as a mammary, child-feeding organ. Couples with doubts must therefore be reassured about the effects of breast-feeding on the woman. Breast-feeding followed by gradual weaning will produce less longterm change than sudden weaning at the outset.

Genuine contra-indications to breast-feeding are rare and include specific diseases in the mother (such as tuberculosis, some kinds of nephritis) and the taking of certain medicines, (such as anti-epilepsy drugs). Very rare cases of breast-milk jaundice should not usually be regarded as a contra-indication. The problem of insecticides may become a cause for concern in the future.

As far as attitudes to feeding are concerned, it is worth singling out the woman who takes a purely scientific approach and will respond only to statistics and arguments based on the composition of various milks. The arguments we would use in support of breast-feeding in this connection are no less important and cannot be reiterated often enough.

Human milk contains 11 grams of protein per litre with a 90% coefficient of utilization, while cow's milk contains 33 grams per litre with a 75% coefficient of utilization. In human milk only one third of the protein content is in the form of casein which coagulates into small flakes and is reduced by the gastric juices to one pH of acidity. Even after diluting to one quarter strength, formula milks contain double the quantity of protein necessary, and this excess leads to additional energy expenditure for digestion and extra work for the liver and kidneys.

Both human and cow's milk contain similar quantities of lipids (fats), but human milk is much richer in unsaturated fatty acids which are vital during the period of growth (particularly for nerve tissue).

Glucosides (sugars) are present in human milk in the proportion of 70 grams per litre, including 8 grams nitric oligosaccharides (glycopeptids which promote the development of the lactic, bacterial intestinal flora peculiar to the nursing baby), and in cow's milk in the proportion 50 grams per litre, exclusively as lactose. At the present time saccharose is used to compensate for the deficit in cow's milk.

However, the differences between human and cow's milk are most evident in their respective hydroelectrolytic composition and osmotic charge. There are four times more mineral salts in cows' milk. In some conditions formula-fed babies may reach the upper limit of urinary concentration. Mother's milk, on the other hand, contains a high percentage of iron in an assimilable form and a better calcium/phosphorus balance.

Finally there are scientific arguments concerning the transfer of maternal antibodies through the milk, although in man, the primates, the rabbit and the guinea pig transfer through the placenta is much more important (unlike the sheep, cow, horse and pig).

It must be pointed out that the formula milks now advertised are becoming increasingly close in chemical composition to mother's milk, although they can never be as good. The danger of these new milks may be all the greater since they may be used to dissuade women from breast-feeding and to promote the idea of feeding as no more than a giving of nourishment.

Some readers may think this discussion of breast-feeding somewhat tedious, but we consider it an important subject, because in the best cases breast-feeding remains the only way of reducing the ill effects of that neo-natal kidnapping committed in technologically advanced maternity units.[1]

---

[1]The effect of breast-feeding on the emotional development of the mother-child pair is explained by recent discoveries in endocrinology. Secretion in the mammary gland is triggered off by hypophysial prolactin and there is reason to believe that this same hormone also triggers mothering behavior in a more general way. Injections of prolactin into mice, even pre-pubescent animals, produces nest-building activity. To suppress milk before artificial feeding, hormonal products which inhibit the release of hypophysial prolactin are given and there is no stimulation of the nipple by sucking, so that the neurohormonal reflex

Obviously a good mother will still be good enough even if she is restricted to artificial feeding. A lack of rigidity, the way the bottle is given and respect for the rhythm of each baby may be more important than the composition of the actual milk. Quoting Plato's Symposium and Christ's Last Supper, the dietician Tremolières reminds us that feeding is also a way of joining us to the human community: 'It is a sin against the flesh to reduce it to a form of hygiene, a functional activity.' The attitude towards feeding the newborn is part of the overall atmosphere in any maternity unit. There is a tendency to overlook the noise level, to disregard the way in which feeding times impose their own rhythm. In our utopian unit, we play discreet and almost imperceptible background music. At the moment I am listening to Rimsky-Korsakov's *Hymn to the Sun,* but it could equally well be a Hindu chant, Saint-Säens' *Swan,* Schumann's *Traümerei* or Liszt's *Liebestraum.*

which might produce secretion of prolactin will not be activated. Obviously we should be careful to avoid hasty extrapolation from the animal world to the human species. Indeed, on an individual level, human behavior appears less dependent on hormonal fluctuation than animal behavior, although eminently influenced by cultural factors. Even so, the spread of bottle-feeding, i.e. the suppression of prolactin secretion in a large percentage of women, should be regarded as cause for concern.

Chapter Nine
THE PEOPLE WHO COME TO US

We have described our own progress from emotional response to reasoned argument. We have shown how an understanding of Leboyer totally changed the attitudes and atmosphere generally associated with obstetrics departments. We have pointed out that birth without violence is not a method, a technical modification which can be rapidly and easily assimilated by means of some indeterminate reform. It is a development in concepts; a revolution.

Any description of the current climate in our unit, however, would be incomplete without some reference to those women and men who do most to make this revolution possible. Who comes to our unit? What kind of people are they?

We can divide them roughly into two types. Most couples choose the place for geographical reasons. There are no other maternity units in our local catchment area of about 45,000 inhabitants. These people form a representative cross-section of society. They are country people, manual workers, business, professional and public service staff. These 'indigenous' women do not usually find anything unusual in our unit, although women with several children find it very changed. Those having their first child who know little about prevailing conditions elsewhere appear to assume that our unit is the norm.

Then there are those couples who come to the unit from choice, even from considerable distances, and these represent an extraordinary variety of lifestyles, cultural and

social backgrounds and aspirations. The very diversity of
their origins and motivations has brought to light the
hundreds of ways in which Leboyer can be read and his
message received, and their wide-ranging backgrounds
may provide a basis for various kinds of research. For
example, in 1975 total prematurity figures were 18 per
550 births. All these occurred among women living in our
catchment area. There were none among the 75 or so
women who came to us from some distance who had
emphasized the importance they attached to the
atmosphere in which birth took place from the beginning
of their pregnancies. Early in 1976 we had our first premature birth in a 'motivated' mother, which coincided day
for day with the date on which the father left for
Guatemala. There is clearly a considerable gap between
medical logic and the logic of the significant.

Some of the women who come to us live in the great
industrial conurbations. Conscious of how adversely they
themselves have been affected by the anonymity and
boredom inherent in our present standardized existence,
they dream of a different, kindly world in which their
children can be born. Unable to satisfy the two basic psychological needs for identity and stimulation, they place all
their hopes in Leboyer's message. They have set out
deliberately to look for a maternity unit with a human face.
In them we can see the expression of a certain kind of
political awareness.

Couples from various socio-cultural backgrounds, of
whom one partner has undergone psychoanalysis or
analytic psychotherapy, come to our unit for different
reasons. In their case, the search for a particular
atmosphere in which to establish relations with the
newborn appears to be part of an attempt to redefine

interpersonal relations as a whole. Some of them have thus experienced pregnancy, delivery and the postpartum period as a time of 'development' despite possible fears that pathological phenomena might reappear.

There are women who have been classified as high-risk pregnancies during early monitoring in high-technology maternity units. In desperation they turn to the kind of unit where medical arguments yield to other forms of reasoning.

Militant supporters of family planning and similar movements have for some time considered the effects on the mother-child relation of planned conception and are concerned about the usual conditions of birth. Clearly it will never be possible to define pregnancy as 'wanted' or 'unwanted' in absolute terms. That would be oversimplifying things and underestimating the importance of ambivalence. An ambivalent attitude to the unborn child is quite natural provided it is not taken to extremes. Emotions do not deal in black and white. In this context it is interesting to read the birth announcement written for 'Sylvie', a child born in our unit:

> But should we do more than simply register our impotence before a society which ordains the very gestures we should use to educate our children, and a child who will doubtless herself refuse to be simply a reflection of ourselves?
>
> Certainly we should.
>
> From the heart of those class contradictions which run through us (and Sylvie with us) and mold our vision of the world, history, life and death, we will give birth to the new man, the collective man, stripped of private property, 'resuscitated'.

Whatever forces affect our daily lives, there is a continuous choice to be made between the old, crumbling world of dying capitalism and the fraternal, united struggle of peoples for their freedom.

Joined to Sylvie not by the bonds of blood alone, but even more by our political will to give life beyond the actual moment of birth, we are no less deeply different from her and will soon find ourselves in constant confrontation.

Not with the superficiality of the family unit, nor in the polarity between parents and child which reflects a so-called generational conflict, but in a process of mutual education, a dialectical resolution of the contradictions which will both set us apart and bring us together and which will reflect in their own way the dynamics of life.

Child, you were not born by chance.

Child, we desired your arrival.

Child, we are giving you life on this day in the history of humanity as it marches across the contradictions which are the backswing of its forward movement.

Child, we will not 'let you live'[1] We are not producing you as if you were some human residue to be kept, dare we say it, alive, just because a male cell once fertilized an egg.

Child, you were born quite especially in the middle of the fight we, your parents, are fighting, a fight in which we will help you grow as you will change us.

Child, you were born specially in the midst of our own parents, relatives, friends and comrades.

You, too, parents, friends, comrades, you will not 'let this child live'. For then this birth would be simply one

[1]This was the slogan of the anti-abortion lobby in France which opposed regalization of abortion.

more occasion, like a marriage, a funeral, on which to eat and drink together, a celebration from which each person goes his separate way when the party is over.

Parents, friends, comrades.

Be more than a friend to Sylvie: be a real comrade. So that through you a breach is made in the walls of that private family life which the old society continually builds around us all. So that through you, Sylvie is really born into the world in the storm wind of history.

We can see from this declaration that the militant supporters of family planning, used to mobilizing popular opinion, may also be linked to those with more explicitly political ideals.

We refer here to the New Left which runs outside the traditional Marxist mainstream and believes change to be the essential word of command; but not change through traditional political activism since economic and political revolution alone may not be enough. The New Left has understood Leboyer. 'To change life', you must change 'everything, straight away'. We will not change life or humanity without first changing the way in which we are born. Political awareness has already penetrated the maternity unit.

The year in which Leboyer's book appeared also saw a new politicization of medicine which probably helped to win a wider public and a greater understanding for his work. As J. C. Polack observes, since the Ancient Greeks medicine had formed 'an island in the ocean of political causes'. But now, ever since the radical re-thinking of most of our social and political institutions since the 'sixties, medical ideology, institutions, instruments and results are being questioned as well. In France the GIS or *Groupe Information Santé* has been formed as a forum for those who regard their work as part of the class struggle, although not necessarily in the factory or workshop. The doctors within the GIS are well aware that their social position places them on the same side as the dominant and powerful, and they do not deny this; but they reject any form of medicine that turns people into objects and the kind of science which covers up an underlying oppression. Their struggle is against the mystification of technical skill and, as such, embraces the promotion of birth without violence.

It is worth emphasizing that at the very moment when Leboyer was writing his book, Ivan Illich was also questioning the good intentions of the English-speaking medical world in an outspoken and deliberately shocking article in the *Lancet* on the subject of *Medical Nemesis*. The author of *Tools for Conviviality* stands as a symbol of misgivings about the medical world and the institutionalization of human life from the cradle to the grave. He sees the most significant impact of medical and hospital provisions as being the iatrogenesis of anxiety, pain, chronic ill-health and maladjustment. Any society able to reduce professional intervention to a minimum will provide the best environment for good health. Illich's views are also a condemnation of the world-wide imperialism of the technological ideal. The question he continually raises is: where is the dividing line between what every person can do for himself, either by himself or with the help of family and/or friends and what that person requires professional help for? But although Illich discusses sickness, death and the medical colonization of everyday life in some detail, he had no opportunity to examine the usual conditions of birth in our advanced societies. And yet surely, turning pregnancy into an illness and delivery into a surgical operation is the most obvious and extreme form of medicalizing everyday life?

Anyone who has spent any time in our unit will have seen how many supporters of ecological movements are now joining the ranks of those who protest against the dominant medical ideology. Believing as they do that society has lost control over technology, ecologists have become enthusiastic followers of Leboyer. Through them we have become acquainted with various like-minded movements in France and elsewhere. Dr Shelton's Hygienist Movement in the United States has long taken an interest in delivery and birth. Shelton believes that since all conscious functions are normally pleasant, delivery should be a pleasure, an orgasmic experience rather than an occasion for suffering. He deplores the fact that professional obstetricians intervene so frequently to disturb deliveries which without their help would most probably be normal (*Dr Shelton's Hygienic Review,* June 1969). In the great majority of cases, all the obstetrician has to do is to receive the newborn child and to perform various simple tasks which were once the province of the woman's neighbors, or of the new mother herself in many so-called primitive tribes. The documentation on delivery compiled and distributed by Shelton's disciples is particularly interesting for the serious comments it contains on the respective advantages and disadvantages of various obstetrical positions. There are vehement arguments against the supine position.

The fact that Leboyer's message has attracted non-violent communities might seem part of the evidence needed. He has, after all, reminded us of the words of Lao-tzu:

When he is born man is soft and weak; in death he

becomes stiff and hard. The ten thousand creatures and all plants and trees while they are alive are supple and soft, but when they are dead they become brittle and dry. Truly, what is stiff and hard is a companion of death; what is soft and weak is a companion of life. Therefore, the weapon that is too hard will be broken, the tree that has the hardest wood will be cut down. Truly, the hard and mighty are cast down; the soft and weak set on high.

In fact, supporters of non-violence see it chiefly as a strategy, as the method most likely to bring about a social revolution because it has the threefold power of mobilizing and reinforcing the exploited (without turning them into tyrants), of weakening and demoralizing the establishment and of winning over the silent majority. Non-violence is basically a defensive strategy which, once organized, provides a shield against all attack. At the present time its supporters appear more concerned with and committed to conscientious objection than the conditions of birth. But that can easily be remedied. (Indeed, since the first edition of this book the French journal *Combat Non Violent* has devoted several articles to birth.)

Despite appearances,
nothing changes.
And it is still from the East
that the light comes to us.
Without Sw. and without India
this book would never have been written.
The idea itself
would not have come to me.

Those who seek 'truth' and transcendental reality outside rationalist western philosophies, outside dogmatic religion or social and conventional morality, are following the same path as Leboyer. We refer here to the various schools of eastern meditation, such as Zen. During 'spiritual discussion' the disciple has to find answers to certain questions without thinking too much about them. Experts in yogic philosophy despise the intellect. They see the ceaseless movement of cerebral thought as a mist which hides the divine from us. It is in the sources of pleasure, not thought, in our own bodies that we can reach the creative principle of the world. It is through corporal techniques that we can perceive that absolute of which we are but fragmentary manifestations. Without the influence of India, Leboyer would not have taught us the first language of skin against skin, that skin from which all the other sensory organs are derived.

Leboyer is both mystic and poet, and it is his poetry which has made him comprehensible to many. They will be afraid that our attempt to interpret Leboyer may also destroy his original message through rationalization. That his words are poetical there can be no doubt:

He bends,
he bends down,
he bows,
he is humble.
He kisses the earth.
He submits to Her.
And in so doing, closing his body, his chest,
he grows empty.
He dies . . .
and without breath, he takes on again the posture of that child-like state before he was born.
Then, having bowed low, having touched with his forehead She who bears him, feeds him, to whom he

will one day return.
He is ready to be reborn.
He stands,
he stretches.
His back opens out, expands.
Air fills him.
And upright, his eyes to heaven, caught by the light,
borne by its inspiration, he trembles, feeling the force
which invades him.
Yes, that is prayer.
That is the short, the long road which goes from the
depth of the waters, crosses the earth, the air
to fly on high.
That is the hard road that Life has run and that every
being re-runs as it is born.
Do we pray as we run?
Does it take only one second to be born?

Like all poets Leboyer stands on the fringes. In opposition
to that blend of science and power which is the great
phenomenon of modern times, he raises poetry as an
anti-scientific, anti-political force. By making poetry of our
everyday experience, he reminds us that poetry is an
attitude to things, an intellectual and moral condition, a
way of seeing and behaving in the face of the world.
Leboyer's distinction is that he recreates the poetical, non-
rational state of mind and uses it in a context where it has
long since been rejected. Custom has such a strong hold
that it will take some time to learn how to rediscover this
'paralogical' condition in the labor room. By his surrealist
approach Leboyer retains a continuous sense of the
marvellous; he gives joy by stimulating that perpetual
astonishment of anyone discovering the real world; he
awakens a new vision by disordering the mind.

Only the baby remains.

That ancient, eternal and illusory division between the watcher and the watched has ended.

All that remains is this child whom we contemplate. Not with what we know about him, what we have learned, what we have been told, what has been read to us. We contemplate him such as he is.

We look at him. Or rather we allow him to flow into us. Without reference. Without prejudice. In all innocence. In all newness.

We become him!

The helpmate has become a newborn child again.

One thing is common to all those whom Leboyer has brought together, the family planners, the politically conscious, the opponents to medical ideology, ecologists, the hygienists, the non-violent, the mystics and the poets: and that is a need to understand humanity, a desire to change life.

Birth Without Violence has also given food for thought to those whose training or professions are concerned with the future of humanity. Since November 1974 we have participated in discussions on birth without violence with students at teacher training colleges. Certain teachers, particularly those in nursery education, have been especially receptive to Leboyer's message. Similarly we have noted an immediate response in trainee paediatricians and practising children's nurses. It was this that gave us the idea of forming an alternative school for midwives.

Many psychoanalysts instantly understand Leboyer. Some have paved the way for him, others followed the same route. Many of those engaged in the exploration of the unconscious find that *Birth Without Violence* comes as a self-evident truth, almost like a memory rediscovered during analysis, familiar yet hitherto blurred. In appreciating Leboyer, psychoanalysis has undoubtedly benefited from current trends in thinking on sexuality, turning away from phallocentrism to matricentrism. Woman no longer defines her position in relation to man, but in relation to the matrix, the mother. She is not a man from whom something is missing. Similarly the child is not a substitute phallus but the objectification of the matrix. Thus it is man who becomes redefined as a woman in whom something is lacking. He is dominated by the longing for pregnancy, his anxieties are those of sterility, not of castration. Erection is a desire to attain the creative world of the woman. These theories would appear to be confirmed by male resistance to vasectomy and by the father's need for activity in the delivery room. In the face of birth, man questions his own role. It may be that these ideas will help to explain the many useless gestures generally performed at labor.

At the time when Groddeck was first developing these matricentrist theories, Otto Rank was writing about the trauma of birth. Rank's ideas do not contradict Groddeck's; more often than not they complement them. When Rank asks why our whole attitude to the world is dominated by the male viewpoint, he does not conclude, as Adler does, that this is due to the social undervalueing of woman, but he believes on the contrary that it is the manifestation of the early repression by which men seek to deprecate woman, to deny her any social and intellectual value because of her association with the birth trauma.

As we attempt to bring back to consciousness the repressed and primitive memory of the birth trauma, we believe that we are revalidating woman by throwing off the curse attached to her genital organs.

At the present time psychoanlysis is also examining the significance of the placenta and 'the myth of fusion'. This believes that our civilization has always neglected the placenta as mediator. By forming a barrier between mother and child the placenta clearly interferes with the myth of primordial unity. According to Bernard This, Rank's one-sided view of the birth trauma merely reinforces this myth and ultimately denies the father any function since his part is not evident at birth. Bernard This also believes that pain in labor supports the myth of fusion: 'You can see that this child is my flesh and my blood and my life since it hurts me so badly when I have to part with it.'

The resolute wish to receive the child as a 'diminished, incomplete, deaf and blind' being, the massacre of the innocents which is a daily performance in our maternity units, may also be related to that dream of fusion we all share.

Chapter Ten
DISCUSSIONS AND DELIBERATIONS

'It may be that traditional man has already been
doing too much and thinking too little for centuries.'
HEIDEGGER

In a 'convivial' unit, where the dividing lines between the
caring and the cared-for tend to disappear along with the
rigid classification of skills, where people come from all
walks of life, and where attempts are being made to build
a true community within a pleasant framework, the climate
is right for discussion, research and rethinking. The topics
we have covered are so diverse that we may now present a
better picture of them by jumbling them together in the
same way that they have occurred to us.

Before going any further there is one statement to be
made: the movement toward birth without violence or
gentle birth is irreversible. Any woman who has
experienced the new climate, either as a mother or as a
witness, will find the current atmosphere in most maternity
units today intolerable in the future. This is also true of
obstetrical staff who have become familiar with the
atmosphere and actions described by Leboyer. They will
find it impossible to work happily in a more orthodox set-
up. It is true that some young nurse-midwives trained in
the official colleges adapt quickly and easily to work in our
unit. Even so, there is a considerable temptation to train
our own staff here, possibly to establish an alternative
school for nurse-midwives and selectively for paediatric
nurses; and we have gone some way to realizing this

project. By saying that the move towards birth without violence is irreversible, we are emphasizing its enormous importance, whether or not the obstetrical profession has understood Leboyer. Surely though, his message was meant for them as well? 'After all this,' he wrote, 'I can say only one thing: Try.'

In fact, many obstetricians have listened to his pleading and appear to be aware of its importance, if only subconsciously. They have expressed their negative views with unusual unanimity in popular women's magazines (e.g. *Elle*, March 1974). The majority focus their attacks on the idea of delivery taking place 'in the dark' where it would be impossible to observe the code of safety it has taken so long to construct. To quote one clinical professor, a member of the Academies of Medicine and Surgery in France:

I believe that we have enough real problems to solve during labor without indulging in ritualistic daydreams leading to activities of more than questionable usefulness. There is no doubt that to be born must be a disagreeable experience for a child, although it is hard to extrapolate from our own psyche to that of the fetus ... It seems to me that delivering babies in the dark must be a gamble when it is still difficult enough while we can see what we are doing. And then to receive the baby in a bath is merely to delay its departure from the liquid environment. It will have to come out sooner or later. I find the whole business quite superfluous since, as you so rightly say, it deliberately directs the attention of the obstetrician toward tasks which may well distract them from the essentials of their skill. I am grateful to you for having brought matters to a head ...

We have also read the following words from a former head of a medical faculty:

> If there is one dangerous and painful moment for the baby during labor it is not the moment of the first cry or the first breath but the prolonged phase of uterine contraction, the engaging of the head and its passage through what may be a narrow pelvis ... If we are to reduce the number of birth complications in France, which is still high, we must train plenty of gynaecological obstetricians and midwives; I do not believe that subdued lighting, warm baths and 'making maternal love' constitute the first step in training new French obstetricians.

And, speaking of the newborn in thermodynamic terms, the former head of an obstetrics and gynaecology department has written:

> The suggestion that an absence of violence can only occur in a situation which threatens proper oxygenation is potentially harmful. Everyone knows that the quality of fetal oxygenation during the first minute of life will affect the quality of the future human being. At the age of sixteen you would rather have been born oxygenated and screaming than anoxic and caressed. Village idiots are sometimes happy as well.

To sum up, we shall quote the essentially Parisian viewpoint of a former head of the gynaeology faculty in Paris, as expressed in the women's press:

> Just a few lines to say congratulations on your courage and clear thinking in condemning the retrograde and dangerous methods of a member of my profession ... your fight against the fashionable trend towards 'natural

childbirth' does you credit. These lunatics forget that maternal mortality has fallen from 1 in 1000 a few decades ago to 1 in 5000 now ... not to mention the infant mortality rate where progress has been even more extraordinary. Thank you for your strong and intelligent protest.

These initial criticisms were unequivocal in their meaning: Leboyer's words are dangerous; they will increase the figures for maternal and perinatal mortality. What the authors of these attacks did not see was that Leboyer was simply drawing our attention to the dual role of the nurse-midwife or obstetrician: first, to ensure that the baby passes from life *in utero* to life in the air without damage to the vital organs, in particular the brain which must receive sufficient oxygen at all times; and second, to do nothing which might gratuitously impede the establishment of the parent-child relationship, hamper the first organizational phase of the newborn child's libidinal life. This second aspect is most often neglected.

After some deliberation, based on our own experience, we are convinced that these two roles are entirely reconcilable and not in the least contradictory. Indeed, they are complementary. It does not seem at all dangerous to us to concentrate a little more on the child being born and perhaps a little less on the way in which the woman is controlling her contractions. Obviously, if a baby is born in acute distress, e.g. following inhalation of amniotic fluid, any respiratory or metabolic difficulties must be appropriately treated by aspiration, ventilation and so on in order to minimize neurological damage. Some obstetricians appear to ignore the fact that unnecessary crying and thrashing about on the baby's part will only lead to even greater oxygen consumption, which does not help intra-cerebral blood circulation at all; whereas skin contact and massage stimulate the respiration, promote brain function and reduce the additional need for oxygen created by prolonged crying.

The change in perinatal mortality figures in our unit would appear to speak for itself. To answer any fears expressed by Parisian obstetricians:

- up to 1 October 1962, 29 deaths per 1000 births;
- for the 1000 births before 1 October 1972, 17 deaths,
- for the 2000 births before 1 July 1975, 14 per 1000,
- for the 1000 births before 1 July 1975, 12 deaths;
- for the 1000 births before 1 April 1976, 10 deaths (including a still birth at home when the mother had stayed at the unit for observation after labor).

During this last period we also had 7.6% caesarians, while the post of a full-time medical anaesthetist remained unfilled.

Following the initial, immediate, violent and vehement protests, there came a second wave of more considered and subtle reactions to Leboyer, this time in medical periodicals. In one of our outstanding provincial medical journals, for example, a gynaecologist-obstetrician of some standing wrote a long analysis of Leboyer's work in which irony appeared to be the dominant note. His, however, was the viewpoint of the gynaecologist-obstetrician. In the same edition of the same journal his wife wrote an article putting forward 'the point of view of the mother'. By simply quoting various carefully selected extracts from Leboyer, this woman expressed her sensitivity to his poetry and her awareness of its importance. More than anything else, her piece was a powerful exhortation to read Leboyer.

Finally, in a professional journal with a nationwide readership, a medical college principal of unquestioned ability and learning offered his ideas, in a way which led us, too, to examine the true significance of Leboyer's book. This eminent obstetrician summed up the position quite simply: 'Why this universal opposition to a book which is as anodine as it is poetic, and not only from doctors but also from women's papers which are usually knowledgeable about psychology and not above telling fairy-tales to judge from their horoscopes?' Or, in other words, 'All things considered, there is no doubt that Doctor Leboyer is slightly way out, but not very dangerous. Other people in much higher positions, both in France and elsewhere, are no less way out, but infinitely more dangerous.' The author of this article regards Leboyer's work as 'a book about obstetrics'. When it comes to Leboyer's practical suggestions, however, he remembers the advice to dim the lights and avoid bustle in the delivery room, to delay cutting the cord and to give a warm bath, but there is no reference to the first language of skin against skin, the firm, slow visceral massage which many mothers will spontaneously give the baby when the atmosphere is right. He ignores the essence.

This omission is extremely significant. Both in adult-child and inter-adult relations, the importance of massage as a means of non-verbal communication and of transmit-ing a sense of well-being is usually neglected. Reich's idea of massage as a method of breaking down the 'corporal breast-plate' has not been widely publicized. Whatever form they may take, it is evident from the criticisms of

Leboyer that convincing the obstetricians alone will not be enough to raise the general consciousness and provoke condemnation of the present conditions of birth. Indeed we are hopeful that there will be a change in attitude among some of the medical teaching profession whose horizons have hitherto been limited by the introduction of modern technology and the battle against perinatal mortality.

The ability of obstetricians to misread the real meaning of Leboyer's work, possibly because they have given him only a cursory reading, would appear to be shared by an eminent perinatologist. When Jean Lacouture asks the barefoot mandarin in Minkovsky's book of that title about the methods claimed to suppress the child's cry at birth, he replies, 'the theories of which you speak, which are developed in a recent book, consist of several aspects. There is the totally ridiculous idea that the child must not cry at birth, while everyone knows that with that first cry comes the beginning of the first breath. That is ignorance of physiology. Afterwards, a lack of crying in the normal child – I am not speaking of sick or mentally handicapped children – is evidence of a certain equilibrium.' If this is a reference to *Birth without Violence*, then Leboyer's actual words have been overlooked:

At the risk of being tedious, we must return yet again to the baby's cry – the cry that was our point of departure.
'Must the baby cry?'
This question is of paramount importance. Too much is at stake here to risk misunderstandings.
The answer is clear and simple: 'Yes, the child must cry.' And it is essential that the cry be what is called 'a good cry'. Resonant, vigorous. A clear cry in which the baby's whole body participates.

If the child is born stunned, if it is limp, if it is waiting instead of crying, every step should be taken *instantly* to produce a sharp, satisfactory cry.

This much is obvious – and there should be no possibility of misunderstanding.

In the same way, if the child coming into the world is being strangled by its umbilicus, we should not hesitate for an instant to cut it and set the baby free.

One question we have asked ourselves, and which people have often asked us, is why are obstetricians so hostile? There are many possible contributory reasons.

The propagation of obstetrical methods, techniques and attitudes, like the dissemination of medical knowledge in general, is controlled by a number of large teaching hospitals which are regarded as the authorities on the subject. This is just another aspect of the move towards centralization which reaches into all areas of society and which Paul Goodman condemns as humanly stultifying. In France, some administrative 'bosses' have publicly expressed a desire for government-controlled perinatology.

Obstetrics departments are run by men who, as males, lack anything more than a rudimentary ability to know by emotional integration, which women enjoy through their maternal instinct, whether or not they are actual mothers.

Obstetricians are for the most part specialists in gynaecology and obstetrics, i.e. they concentrate on the woman. Paediatric obstetricians would probably approach the problem from a different angle.

Obstetricians have made great efforts to assimilate the applications of modern technology. They have allowed themselves to be overwhelmed and intoxicated by this technology and by their pride in themselves as technicians, forgetting that they must be more than technicians. They do think of the child but in 'thermodynamic' terms. In this they are simply part of a general twentieth-century tendency for medical ideas to become blunted by technological intoxication.

For, like most of our contemporaries, obstetricians are technology-mad. This means that before tackling any human problem, they remove all its emotional content in order to strip away their own uncertainties and residual anxieties.

Obstetricians are not aware of their dual role: to monitor the conditions of birth but also to ensure that these conditions are right for the establishment of the mother-child relationship.

Some people believe that many obstetricians themselves had a difficult birth which would explain both their vocation and their traditional behavior towards the newborn. As we have mentioned, Bernard This believes that the myth of primordial unity, the dream of fusion which we all share, lies behind the deliberate desire to receive the newborn child as though it were an invalid.

Obstetricians have not realized that by concentrating more on the child, they would be working towards a reduction in neo-natal mortality and morbidity.

Just as they have ignored the harm done by the propagation of such concepts as high-risk pregnancies which turn labor into a drama, so too have obstetricians been blind to the favorable effect Leboyer's book has had on the general public. Many women who previously had no desire to be mothers in the world in which they lived, have come to want children in the world Leboyer shows them.

Leboyer is a creator, and his creation disturbs existing

institutions. That is why he is rejected by those at the top. Birth without violence is not a *modus operandi* which can be introduced alongside existing methods. It demands the reorganization of every maternity unit.

It is possible that some people object on principle to the idea of birth without violence, since, like Spitz, they believe that frustration is an important factor in learning and development. But all Leboyer is asking is that we should not increase the pressure of frustration and displeasure to which nature already relentlessly submits us from the moment we are born.

Some people interpret the need certain adults feel to welcome newborn babies in a non-violent way as an attempt to eliminate their own fears of castration.

In fact, the objections of obstetricians to Leboyer can only be examined in relation to the characteristics of our society as a whole. In a consumer society where human relationships are bound by the laws of the market-place, it would be extremely surprising if the sensations experienced by the fetus or newborn baby aroused very much interest. Leboyer goes beyond the purely medical and confronts problems which are socio-cultural, philosophical and political. In this sense his work is shocking. The attacks on him are reminiscent of the censure to which Freud and Reich were subjected in their day.

The overall restraint we try to achieve often gives rise to thought and discussion about the perennial human need for activity during labor. The history of obstetrics sometimes looks like a catalogue of futile and dangerous exercises dreamt up to 'facilitate' labour. It is worth describing some of these as examples to show how universal the need for activity has been. The following quotations from H. de Lalung's book *L'Accouchement à travers les ages et les peuples*, begins with one of the most representative exercises, that of Hippocratic succession (a method of shaking):

> The woman is placed on a firm bed lying on her back. A wide band of fabric or a flexible belt is passed round her chest, under her armpits and attached to the bed. Her arms are tied down in the same way. The legs are spread and the feet bound by straps. When the woman in labor has been positioned thus, two bundles of dry, bendy wood or anything that will have the same effect, are placed so that when the bed is raised vertically its feet do not touch the ground. At the same time the woman is told to hold onto the bed with her hands, without resting her head on it, so that her feet will bear the weight of her body and she will not slide off. Once this has been done and the bed raised vertically, the bundles of wood are placed under the feet of the bed so that the connecting crossbar does not touch the ground when it is shaken but rests on the wood. Two men, one on each side of the bed, will then lift it in unison and drop it on the bundles of wood whenever the woman has pains.

This kind of shaking was used for 'normal' labor. In cases of prolonged or difficult labor, Hippocrates had suggested another method:

> Spread a sheet under the woman who should lie on her back. Wrap both arms and both legs in a piece of linen. Two women will take hold of the legs and two others of the arms, then grasping firmly, shake the woman at least ten times. They will then place the woman on the bed with her head down and her legs raised and letting go the arms, all four of them will

shake the legs, jerk the shoulders several times and finally throw the patient back onto the bed so that, thus shaken, the fetus will adopt a different position inside the breadth of her and will be able to travel in a regular fashion.

Albucasis, a 12th century Arabic doctor, advised sitting the patient on a chair with her feet raised: 'You will then shake the seat on the ground, holding the woman so that she does not fall off.' He also recommends administering 'an injection of mucilage of fenugreek and oil of fumitory to induce sneezing with hellebore and to squeeze the abdomen.'

Lalung also tells how Arab midwives energetically massaged the belly and roughly compressed the abdomen with anything they had to hand. Sometimes the midwife would stand on the large plank of wood used for making couscous; others would place on the woman's belly the millstones used for grinding barley and, if presentation was abnormal, roll the woman on the ground. In the Atlas Mountains midwives pressed the woman's belly with their heads and squeezed her round the waist with their hands. In Russia, massage was replaced by the use of the jar. This involved throwing a piece of burning tow into a sandstone jar to make a kind of giant cupping glass which was then applied to the woman's belly. Among the Mongolians, a female bystander would stand on the woman's shoulders and shake her violently, both women hanging onto the tentpeg. Siamese women were hung by their armpits to a rope while one or sometimes two assistants pulled rhythmically at the wretched patient's belly. In Annam the midwife or 'bamu' massaged the vulva with a circular motion, while in India the midwife dilated the vulval orifice by inserting both clenched fists. Among a number of

African people the woman was ordered to pull at a rope or blow into a calabash. If labor was prolonged, the woman was placed on the bottom of a cauldron and, as she clung to the tripod beneath it, an assistant passed a piece of cloth round her belly and then pulled it as hard as he could, supporting his feet on the small of the woman's back. In Loango, the woman is laid on her stomach and trampled on. If necessary the mouth and nose are stopped up so that the wretched woman will struggle and thus hasten delivery. All these exercises are frequently accompanied by drum beating. The Mexicans use a combination of dilatation, massage, compression and shaking. The 'partera' dilates the vulva and massages the abdomen, while the 'tendera' stands behind, squeezes the woman's belly and shakes her violently. Although walking around is often recommended, in Bermuda the walking becomes a positive race around the room. There are even women to beat the patient if she stops. If she falls, the midwives pick her up and trample on her belly to make the baby come out. Quite recently it was still common practice in certain villages in the Auvergne to put chickens on the woman's abdomen so that the scratches their feet produced would accelerate labor.

There is no need to go into the 'cares' lavished on the newborn baby. Only a few decades ago any baby which appeared at all stunned might be subjected to beatings while hung by the feet, vigorous rubbing, sprinkling with alcohol or ether and alternate hot and cold baths.

It is difficult to make a complete break with the past. That is why we have a museum in our unit to display obsolete instruments, in particular forceps. There are scissor-shaped forceps, forceps like tongs, some large and some small. Over the last ten years we have had no occasion whatever to use them. Why do we consider them obsolete? Malinas has provided the definitive answer to this question by likening obstetrical mechanics to the passing of an egg through a ring, and by emphasizing the importance of the middle passage. If progress ceases after the upper passage has been breached and the head is engaged, this is often because the baby's head is not rotating correctly. Since rotation is linked to flexion and only a well-flexed head will be able to rotate, then clearly we have to flex the head. But how? Certainly not with forceps. Whether applied symmetrically (by the cheekbones) or asymmetrically (by mastoid and forehead) the forceps will grip in front of the flexion-deflexion axis of the head and the exertion of traction will tend to deflect the head unless head and blades are fitted together by screwing down the forceps, which will also reduce the transverse diameter . . . this is scarcely birth without violence. In many cases incorrect flexion can be corrected by hand. Malinas has a full description of the method:

– wait for the first contraction;
– introduce the hand flat onto the fetal head so that the fingertips are pressing lightly on the forehead and the thumb hooks over the side of the lambdoid (using the right hand if the occiput is to the right and the left hand if it is to the left);
– very gently push back the forehead, asking the patient to push again, and start rotation with the thumb on the edge of the lambdoid suture.

Vacuum extraction by 'ventouse' is much easier. There is no need to exert any force. Once the ventouse is correctly positioned it can be directed rather than pulled in the right direction with total co-operation from the mother. The ventouse is an aid used in a minority of cases and cannot be compared to forceps.

When we talk about our own experience, the questions most often put to us concern the short and medium term future of children born without violence. It would be tempting to refer, by way of reply, to the much-awaited report of Danielle Rapoport who has conducted research into 120 of some 1000 or so children born with Leboyer's help. Rapoport, a psychologist, has measured the development quotient of children aged one, two and three years and has observed that the mean quotient was higher than a control group (106 as opposed to 100). Her researches appear to have brought to light a certain quality in the mother-child relationship: 112 of the 120 children had no difficulty in learning toilet-training and self-feeding. During the period of research the mothers did not seek any advice or consultation from the psychologist. In fact, we should not be in too much of a hurry to equate the conditions in which the children selected by Rapoport were born and the conditions of birth in our unit. The group she studied were 'delivered' by Leboyer who, in our experience, is better able to calm and communicate with the newborn than anybody else. However, their mothers had come to him by chance without having known him beforehand, without being prepared for birth, whereas in our unit many couples have a good knowledge of the place and then go on to 'deliver' the baby themselves. Almost always the mother's hands massage the baby, often assisted by the father, immediately following birth. Exceptionally, a team member on duty will receive the child and, although his or her gestures may appear stereo-typed, the human warmth they transmit will depend on any number of factors.

We have not yet sought any systematic research into the children born in our unit since recent changes. They are still too young and the bulk of the evidence we have about them comes from their mothers, whose objectivity may not be entirely reliable. It will probably be interesting to hear the opinion of school teachers in a few years time. In any case, the evaluation of states of mind hardly lends itself to statistical research, although we have found that certain specific adjectives have been used to describe these children more than others from the very beginning: fearless, for example, happy and vigorous. The following words come from a woman who has several children:

S... was a newborn baby with an extraordinary appetite for and joy in life. He never cried inconsolably in the evenings, for example, as other babies do. He is lovely: right from the beginning he tugged more and seemed stronger than the others; especially in his back. He would suddenly move around so much on the changing table that I could not leave him to go and fetch something. G.... is also marvellous, but I think as a baby he was not quite so happy, although I was entirely positive about him because I was glad that a child had been born after such a long wait.

In several cases we have found that mothers appeared to relate to their children as separate individuals, perceiving them as independent subjects and not merely as objects of possession, or even of love. This is something Leboyer had hoped would happen:

'Mothers must begin to feel:
"I am its mother,"
and not:

"This is my child."
A world of difference lies between the two.
And the whole future of the child.'

It is worth emphasizing some of the 'negative' observations also. As far as we know, there has been no three-month colic or paroxysmic crying among the babies born in non-violent fashion. This curious syndrome is the subject of a recent study by Kreisler, Frain and Soulé. Although it occurs quite frequently and has been recognized for some time, there is little paediatric literature on the subject, possibly because it is basically benign. We find it important both because of the hypotheses which have been advanced to explain it and as an additional aspect of the psychosomatic phenomenon. The syndrome usually appears 8-10 days after birth, i.e. shortly after returning home from hospital. The crying often starts after a feed, when the baby is full, usually in the evening or at night. Before the crying starts and while it continues the baby makes other noises suggestive of hunger pains or digestive troubles. Examination reveals a certain amount of abdominal swelling which can be identified radiologically as gassy distention. In far too many cases, a remedy is sought in alterations to feeding formula or routine, or even to drugs; whereas there are only two ways to comfort the baby: a dummy and rocking. Everything returns to normal without further intervention at about two to three months. This syndrome has not been observed in babies living in communal environments. The interpretation for this condition offered by Spitz is usually lent most credence. Spitz sees growth as being conditioned by a balance between satisfactions and frustrations, so that when it experiences frustration the baby has to develop an auto-erotic compensatory system to ensure it some autonomy. Without the opportunity to develop this system, some organic trouble will emerge.

In this particular case, two series of factors would appear to prevent the system of compensation from establishing itself. The first is characterized by a specific attitude in the mother who tends to alleviate any sign of suffering in the baby by feeding it. This primary, anxious solicitude may be the result of guilt due to unconscious hostility and would presumably manifest itself in a tense and anxious mother who might be over-protective or impatient.

The second involves a predisposed, hypertonic baby who is expressing an aggravated need for instinctual release. Spitz believes that the age at which the symptoms disappear coincides with the appearance of the first responses directed toward other people, to a smile for example, and with the age at which the mind begins to expand, in a release of tension.

Spitz's interpretation is not incompatible with Kleinian hypotheses. By giving the baby food when it needs something else the mother is introjected into the baby as an internalized bad mother whom the child tries to reject by provoking a spasm of pain. Michel Fain has stressed another aspect of the problem which has not been followed up: namely the very great difficulty these mothers have in coping with their anxiety. Whatever their differences, all these interpretations suggest that there is some disturbance in the mother-child relation behind a problem which appears during the baby's early weeks. It is surprising that no reference is ever made to the dreadful additional frustration provoked in maternity units by the way the child is stolen from the mother at birth. After listening to Leboyer, it will surely be impossible to ignore the first hours of life. Three-month colic is typical of the early somatic manifestations which appear to be linked to an imbalance between satisfaction and frustration. In other words, it is the somatic expression of a very early emotional disturbance. Through a study of this syndrome it would be possible to consider the whole of psychosomatic medicine and examine the effects of additional postnatal trauma along with the profound disturbances continually affecting the early organizational stages of the libido. Of course, there are other aspects of psychosomatic pathology in the nursing baby to be studied which might be equally valuable as a means of understanding the psychosomatic phenomenon. An examination of sleep problems, for example, would reveal the importance of the first experiences of frustration and their effect on later phases.

In fact, it is possible to observe insomnia and nightmares in a small baby whose relationship with the mother is now good but was difficult during the immediate post-natal period. However, nights broken by insomnia will lead in their turn to disturbances in the relationship. Too often insomnia of this kind is treated by tranquilizing or somniferous drugs which will again disturb 'the transitional phenomena' and alter the future of 'transitional objects'.

The real question that needs to be asked about the future of these children is what kind of adults they will be. Will they be very special people, capable of enjoying a real emotional life and engaging in significant relationships? Or will they use their ability to socially integrate, adapt, act and take responsibility to mask a fundamental suffering which will become evident sooner or later? Or, to put it more basically, will they have duodenal ulcers, will they be alcoholics or impotent? But then, we should also be asking, will they be potential creators in artistic or scientific fields? This question occurs to anyone who suspects the existence of a close connection between creativity and the ability to play when they see the newborn taking its first bath. It is already learning how to play, and by playing to explore its own body and the world around it in a way which appears to be indistinguishable from sensual pleasure. It has, after all, been suggested that every creative act has a sensual element. To summarize: our hope is to play a part in the development of a convivial society in which every person is given the opportunity to nurture and exercise their own creativity.

Chapter Eleven
SCEPTICISM AND CRITICISM

When we hold discussions within the unit, the people involved are usually agreed in their conviction that the circumstances of birth are vitally important for the future of the individual, or even of the species. When, on the other hand, we talk about these issues outside the unit, for example during question and answer sessions following a screening of the film *Birth*, we often encounter doubts about the importance of Leboyer's message and scepticism about the significance of the first hours following birth.

The following are examples of the kinds of question we are asked:

Surely the additional postnatal trauma induced by artificial means is negligible compared to certain kinds of acute fetal distress aggravated by anoxia (lack of oxygen) and complications in labor such as constriction-ring dystocia or chronic fetal distress from hypoxia (insufficient oxygen) and complications in pregnancy such as kidney disease, prolonged pregnancy and so on.

To this we reply that these pathological conditions occur only in a minority of cases; that, as perceptive observers, the obstetrical staff are there to anticipate them; that, when they do occur, every possible technological assistance is given; and, whatever the physiological or thermodynamic condition of the baby, any gratuitous action likely to disturb its initial sensory, motor and relational experiences will be damaging.

What is the use of preparation for birth if the baby is born prematurely and then separated from its mother over a long period?

It is never possible to anticipate premature birth in individual cases, although there is always a statistically calculable risk that it may occur. We find that the best way to prevent prematurity is to prepare women so that they experience pregnancy as a happy event, not as an illness.

When premature birth does occur it is often possible to place the incubator by the mother's bed and the mother herself can soon learn how to do the job generally performed by the paediatric nursing staff. Even so, some very premature babies have to be kept in special units, and in these cases the separation of mother and baby over several weeks is always a cause for concern, especially when they are unable to stay in the same building.

Again, we would urge a rapid change in the way that premature baby units are organized once any fear of infection that excludes the mother has passed. It seems likely that the research undertaken by people like Marshall Klaus in the United States and Irene Lézine in France will have beneficial practical efects.

Is preparation for birth useful or counter-productive when the pregnancy ends in a caesarian?

Obviously caesarian section is always a last resort, but couples do understand that more than anything else birth without violence is an atmosphere which permeates the whole maternity unit. Even when a caesarian is performed we handle the baby in a different way so that we can ensure a non-violent welcome for it, in some cases with the father's help. Ideally, forms of anaesthesia such as epidurals and acupuncture which do not alter consciousness should be used, and we are lucky enough to have an anaesthetist trained in epidural technique. In any case, there is nothing to stop a baby delivered by caesarian from being breast-fed. Birth without violence is important less on the individual than on the collective level, and as much in terms of future generations as the present one. Leboyer's work is not confined to the here and now, alone.

Can bathing the baby so soon after birth lead to infection starting in the umbilicus?

Usually the baby is bathed before the cord is finally cut near the navel. We give the bath in a clean basin kept exclusively for this purpose. Some nurse-midwives add a few drops of antiseptic to the water. We think this unnecessary. However, we do consider it important to completely undress the mother and to ensure that her hands, pubis, abdomen and chest are perfectly clean. Anyone who fears an increased risk of infection can be reassured by our experience. Also, the first bath does not remove the *vernix caseosa* or amniotic grease which covers the fetal skin. One of the advantages of the bath is to channel the extraordinary need of activity of the professionals at the time of first contact between mother and baby.

During her stay at the unit over the next few days, there is nothing to stop a mother bathing her baby every day. This has been our practice since 1963.

Isn't the child exposed to cold as it lies in the mother's arms?

The temperature in the delivery room must be kept sufficiently high. The mother's belly and hands are always warm. Although this is not its chief function, the bath also helps to warm the baby. While it is in the bath we warm a towel to wrap round it. In fact, our staff have become so familiar with the language of the newborn that they would immediately recognize any distress due to cold.

If you lay the baby in its mother's arms, surely delayed cord-cutting will adversely affect the baby's circulation?

Since the physiologists have answered this question in various different ways, we tend to reply that our clinical impression is favorable. In their authoritative work on obstetrical and neo-natal practice, S. G. Babson and R. C. Benson point out that the newborn child's physiology is very adaptable, capable of tolerating the withdrawal or addition of blood without risk. However, early cord-cutting may produce a reduction in the volume of blood circulating in the child which will lead to hypotension and possible constriction of the blood vessels. Ideally, the baby should be left on a level with the placenta until the cord has stopped beating so that a balance of blood pressure and volume can be achieved between the child and the placenta. Other researches have been conducted into different aspects of the child's physiology following early or delayed cord-cutting. Lanzkowsky of Capetown, for example, has shown that up to the age of 3 months haemoglobin levels are higher in infants following delayed cord-cutting. A team in Stockholm has examined the effect of delayed cord-cutting on artery diameter and found that

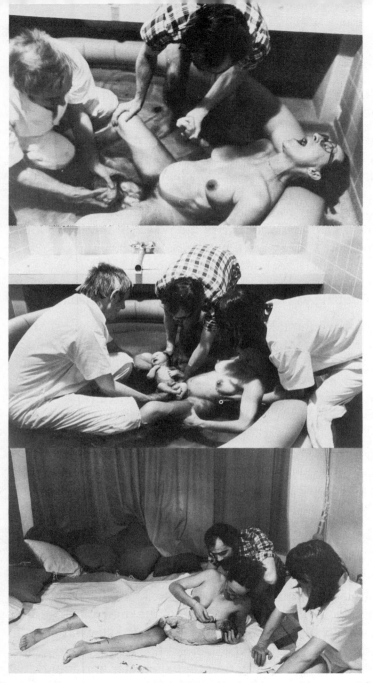

A birth in the warm water pool; Michel Odent lifts the baby out of the water; relaxation in the birthing room Photographs: Jean-Claude Francolon/Gamma

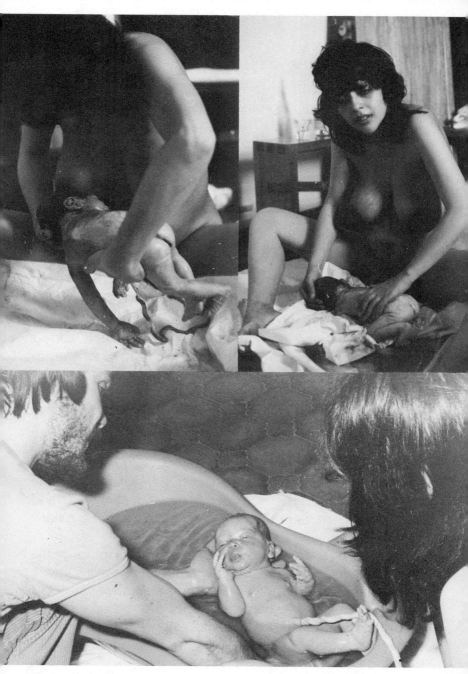

The mother herself handles the newborn. Some babies like a bath. The baby is still attached to its mother by the umbilical cord

arterial circulation to the placenta stops before venous circulation, thereby protecting the baby against any significant loss of blood. There has been less research into the effects on the mother of delayed cord-cutting, although Z. Walsh of Stockholm suggests that early clamping may lead to less loss of blood when the placenta is delivered.

It is worth pointing out that a mother who receives her own baby tends not to remain totally supine and not to place the baby on top of her 'bulge' so that in practice there is no perceptible difference in altitude between the placenta and the baby. In fact, any questions about the risks of infection, cold and haemodynamic conditions related to delayed cord-cutting are usually asked by professionals who have not fully understood what Leboyer is saying. He is not suggesting that we adhere to a series of stereotyped gestures, but simply helping us to think about the baby as a baby and not as an object; to create a particular atmosphere. But every birth will remain a special case. Ultimately, we believe it possible to welcome a newborn baby in subdued light, in silence, to massage its back and to give it a bath without necessarily practising birth without violence, if neither the parents nor the obstetrical staff have grasped the real meaning behind Leboyer's statement that 'without love you will be merely skilful'.

Delivery in water is another way of ensuring gentle transition from the intra-uterine to the aerial environment. If the baby is born under water in this way, any fears about cold or the haemodynamic effects of delayed cord-cutting can be removed. Since the first edition of this book we have acquired the use of small swimming pools. Experience shows that during the first phase of labor, immersion in warm water with eyes closed, in subdued light, and with the ears under water, helps the woman to cut herself off from the outside world and to listen to the instinctive voices within her. In many cases uterine contractions become less painful and more effective. Some women then refuse to leave the water and dreams of underwater birth have become a reality.

There has, admittedly, been very little research into neo-natal physiology, particularly the physiology of the newborn baby still attached to the placenta by the umbilicus. Tchobroutsky confirms this in her study of the initial establishment of respiration. Towards the end of 1975, therefore, a 'group for the study of the newborn' (GEN) was set up in Paris to bring together researchers and practitioners representing many different disciplines (paediatrics, obstetrics, psychoanalysis, psychology, neurophysiology, ethnology, audiology and so on). Clearly Leboyer's thought-provoking and easily understood work inspired the formation of this group.

You suggest that the decline in the number of 'normal deliveries' and the advanced technology of present day maternity units go hand in hand. But surely obstetrical difficulties are characteristic of the human species?

Even among tail-less anthropoids which stand upright, there are never any mechanical difficulties during birth because there is no real pelvic cavity and because the vulval orifice is not off-centre. Moreover, in all the other primates apart from *homo sapiens,* the transverse diameter of the pelvis is always larger than the biparietal diameter of the fetal head, just as the sagittal diameter of the pelvis is larger than the fetal occipitofrontal diameter, in particular among the three great anthropoids (the orangutang, the chimpanzee and the gorilla); while the biacromial diameter (or distance between the shoulders) is always distinctly smaller than the sagittal diameter of the pelvis. What characterizes the species *homo* is the permanent upright stance, the existence of a pelvic cavity with a hollow back, a hollow sacrum, a flat pubic symphysis and an off-centre vulval orifice. In humans the fetal occipitofrontal diameter (120 mm) and the biacromial diameter (120 mm) are larger than the sagittal diameter of the pelvis (105 mm). The fetus travels in a corkscrew motion. In the human species, therefore, even small variations in fetal and maternal dimensions are enough to produce feto-maternal disproportion. Obviously our civilization helps to create such variations by racial mixing and foods too rich in fats and sugars. The plump, chubby-cheeked baby is a human creation. The fact remains, however, that most deliveries should be perfectly normal and advanced technology is itself very often a factor in fetal distress.

Isn't there a risk that birth without violence will spark off a return to home deliveries? (This is the way the question has often been formulated by doctors.)

A historical study of reactions to 'medicalized birth' would show how far the return to home delivery and the behavior of certain alternative communities has been affected by it, particularly in the United States. For our own part we have seen birth without violence as a focal point for attempts to 'de-medicalize' birth within the hospital structure. It is true that non-violent birth has taken place at home in certain parts of France, and these cases have encouraged local obstetricians to reconsider and change their attitudes. Safety in home births or in small rural maternity units would be considerably improved by wider use of small ultrasonic stethoscopes and, in particular, by the introduction of the amnioscope, which permits early detection of fetal distress and thus helps to identify those cases requiring observation in a hospital. The amnioscope is a metal tube with a lighting system which can be powered by ordinary batteries. It is introduced into the cervix and enables medical staff to see the color of the amniotic fluid without rupturing the membranes. Any stain in the fluid is a sign of fetal distress, since a badly oxygenated fetus will empty its intestines of the first faeces or *meconium*. We see the amnioscope as the archetypal convivial tool, simple, cheap and easy to use, as opposed to the elaborate, complicated and expensive tools represented by electronic monitoring systems.

Is birth without violence compatible with the service provided by a large maternity unit where several thousand babies are born each year?

This question is often asked. It is widely accepted that any progress in clinical medicine comes by way of the large hospitals which are well endowed with staff, finance and technology.

Is it possible, then, for the conceptual revolution Leboyer started to be taken up in large maternity units? Obviously when numbers are reasonably low (say two deliveries a day, or 600-1000 a year) each birth can still be a meaningful event. It is equally obvious that a large staff is seldom homogeneous. We believe, therefore, that in the first instance it will be the medium-sized maternity departments that will change as we have. Of course, the atmosphere which now prevails in these units is by no means clear cut. Many hospitals in medium sized towns in

France regard the maternity unit as a second-rank department of no prestige, run by a practitioner who has become an obstetrician by chance, in addition to his main speciality. In some cases the head of department will be a general physician who uses a surgeon for caesarians, more rarely a surgeon himself. In my hospital, for example, the surgical and maternity departments are under one man. We gradually came to realize that the birth of a human being is always a more important and more far-reaching event than many a laborious and costly operation for which the indications were open to doubt. Even in large hospitals obstetrics is always a poor relation in comparison to other special departments. If, as happened in one particular case, it is only possible to build half of a new regional hospital, the departments of surgery, cardiology, resuscitation and gastroenterology, for example, will be set up first while newborn babies continue to make do with the most dilapidated accommodation. This lack of status is not confined to the hospital service; it also applies in the medical career structure. A recent book on doctors by a lecturer in medicine in Paris tells us a great deal. It contains well-written chapters on the general practitioners' well-paid inferno, the specialists' cushioned existence, the surgeons' prestige, the golden road through the teaching hospitals, the humanization of hospitals. There is no mention of the conditions of birth. There is no analysis of the profession of the obstetrician who has to deal with more frequent and urgent emergencies than almost any other specialist. There are, as it happens, two allusions about the obstetrician, both of which are worth quoting. When discussing the prestige of the surgeon, the author recalls an old saying: 'If I had three sons, the most intelligent would be a general doctor, the next a surgeon, the least gifted of the three an obstetrician.' Describing the effects of scarcity in junior surgical posts in hospitals, the author then tells us that future surgeons are forced to join departments on the fringes of their work, such as the obstetrics department.

These few comments on the respective prestige of different medical specialities serve to illustrate the lack of interest in birth betrayed by doctors, administrators, the general public, indeed society as a whole. It would seem that behind this indifference lies a confusion about how to respond when we are confronted with the wretchedness of the baby at the moment of birth. Surely we should be exploring this collective subconscious which exposes our ignorance of the newborn.

Don't you worry that by placing so much emphasis on the conditions of birth you may have overlooked or underestimated the importance of the conditions of conception, the social background to it, the relations between the parents?

To describe a pregnancy as either wanted or unwanted is an oversimplification, as we have already pointed out. In any case, the development of contraceptive techniques and legislation have changed the bases by which we can define pregnancy as 'desired'. Obviously the child can be more or less wanted; but it should be welcomed into the world, whatever the case. In fact, it is arguable that the less love there is at the time of conception, the more destructive, irreversible and definitive will be the consequences of the baby's seizure at birth by the 'dutiful but undelighted' hands of the technician. Research conducted by Irene Lézine and Robson and Moss leads to surprising or alarming conclusions about the behavior of the mother-child pair at birth and the moment when the first manifestation of maternal instinct appears. Robson and Moss found that 34% of women experience neutral or even quite detached feelings for the newborn child and that 7% actually feel negative and aggressive. These figures may be an indication of the destructive effect of birthing practice in most modern maternity units.

Surely mother-love precedes birth. Aren't you overlooking the importance of the intra-uterine life, the mother-child relation before birth?

Obviously the child exists long before birth in the mother's fantasies and imagination, and by becoming part of a language circuit from a very early stage. It is even possible to argue that as soon as a little girl enters into the Oedipal conflict and discovers her external genital organs, she is already foreseeing her own role as a mother and imagining herself a mother as her own mother is. It is also interesting to speculate on the degree to which the development of mother-love during pregnancy may be influenced by a fore-knowledge of how the baby will be received at birth.

Over the centuries there have been endless hypotheses, commentaries and inferences about the relationship between the mother and the fetus *in utero*. Thomas Aquinas claimed that the soul is always thinking, even during sleep and before birth. Pregnant women can relate their own observations of how emotion, rest, exhilirating or calming music affect fetal movement. According to popular tradition maternal emotions have a direct influence on the child, a notion which has given rise to a whole host of beliefs about cravings, birthmarks and malformations. Medical theory has long suggested that influences on the fetus are less direct, with the mother's body acting as intermediary.

Electroencephalography has enabled us to carry out objective comparative studies of cerebral activity in mother and baby and in particular to examine the paradoxical sleep which accompanies the dreaming activity so necessary for creativity. There is evidence that the nocturnal movements of the fetus *in utero* occur during the mother's dreams. Electroencephalography has also highlighted the effects of barbiturates and other drugs used by women towards the end of pregnancy. Some people have traced the origins of language and human intelligence back to the intra-uterine life. Tomatis believes that intra-uterine communication is the cause and origin of our specifically human desire to speak. The fetal sense of hearing is characterized by its functioning within the liquid environment. It is possible to artificially create a similar sense of watery surroundings by passing the sound through electronic filters. Filtered sound can then be used to recreate intra-uterine conditions for a subject and arouse in him a desire for 'the most archaic of relations': that with the mother. These sounds are constructed from the maternal voice which is one of the chief noises the embryo perceives, by filtering it beyond 8000 hertz. Filtered sounds have been used in particular for the treatment of dyslexics and also for schizophrenics. Tomatis believes that the schizophrenic is someone who was not recognized by her or his mother before birth. After a certain number of sessions using filtered sounds, the filtering of the mother's voice is reduced from 8000 to 100 hertz to achieve a kind of sonic delivery. This phase of the cure restores a balance to all those who were unable to hear their mother's voice at the right time. The patient is then able 'in two or three sessions to relive or to experience for the first time that crucial moment of his human existence during which he should have entered the world through his relationship with his mother.'

The heartbeat technique developed by Duran Lopez seeks to release anxiety by a return to the fetal state. Similarly, Hajime Murooka has tried to reproduce the ambiant sound which the baby perceives in the uterus. Feijo claims to have calmed the newborn child by using low frequency sound (less than 2000 hertz) of the kind to which the fetus *in utero* has been sensitized.

Others regard the intra-uterine life as paradise itself. Our whole life then becomes a desire to return to the abundance of the matrix, the organ of our individual paradise, where the paradise of the collective imagination was created. This was the view of Ferenczi, who believed that birth is a catastrophe, a severing of relations with the mother, a passage from the pleasure state to the reality principle.

Certainly Leboyer sees the intra-uterine life as paradisiacal 'To make love is to return to Paradise, it is to plunge again into the world before birth, before the great separation. It is to rediscover the primordial slowness, the blind, all-powerful rhythm of the internal world, of the great ocean,'

At first sight, the child in the womb is sheltered from fundamental frustration. Within the womb any need seems to be immediately answered by satisfaction. This is not to say that suffering is unknown. It has been shown that, when a pregnant woman faces stress, her secretion of 'stress' hormones may be dangerous for the fetus. Indeed Janov claims to have discovered it in certain cases through the primal experience. But, however we view the significance of the intra-uterine life, it will end in a total reappraisal of the parent-child relationship, in a harsh encounter of fantasy and reality. For that is birth, and that is the most important moment. Too often it is the moment of the massacre.

Aren't you overestimating the importance of birth in relation to the wide variety of environments into which the baby will be received when it leaves your unit? What will become of a newborn child received in non-violent fashion if s/he is then deprived of a normal family environment?

To answer this question you have first to define the normal family. Is the over-conformist and conventional family really normal or normalizing? Should we always suppose that the most alienating family environment is a product of the most alienated family? Without knowing what a normal family environment is like, can one validly study the effects of being deprived of it? The usual definition, of course, takes the normal parents to be two people of opposite gender who live together and have biologically created the child; so that when the baby is reared in any other circumstances s/he is deprived of a normal family background. It is true that outside the stereotype there are often all kinds of anomaly: one or both parents may be temporarily or permanently missing, incapable of fulfilling their role; the couple may have emotional or financial problems. We are not suggesting that family breakdown produces no psychological or emotional repercussions. Leboyer expressed the importance of the family context in telling simplicity: 'Cutting the umbilicus at the first cry is the same as withdrawing the hand at the first step.' The effects of separating parents and child and of depriving the baby of a normal family environment have been the subject of many works, including those by Anna Freud, Dorothy Burlingham, Bowlby, Michael Rutter, Bissonnier, Myriam David and Genevieve Appell. Ragot has shed an interesting light on the topic by comparing the anxiety of the void experienced when parachute jumping and the anxieties of the emotional life. He asks whether young children making repeated jumps into the emotional void may not repress their anxiety by a reciprocal conditioned inhibition mechanism and subsequently become incapable of love. It is worth emphasizing just how much research has been done into the reactions of the very young baby to a slackening of or total break in the mother-child bond, while the ways in which this bond is first created by the circumstances of birth are rarely analyzed or even mentioned. In other words, the more spectacular breaks in the parent-child bond attract more attention and usually arouse much more interest than the useless, traditional and apparently unavoidable acts disturbing the first minutes, hours and days of extra-uterine life.

Aren't you underestimating the aims and effects of education? When the child has been helped to develop and achieve over many years by teachers and educationalists, what traces will remain of those few privileged moments at birth?

Nobody will deny the effects of education, although its aims are ill-defined and have changed a good deal over the years. Education has always been subordinate to the prevailing ideology. At one time the common purpose of education was to prepare people for their chief task in life, the fulfilment of God's purpose as revealed to man by religion. It was no mere matter of chance that churches were the largest buildings in medieval Europe. Education, then, urged people to master their baser instincts so that they might please God. Later (and even now in some countries) education became chiefly preparation to serve one's country by building and preserving national unity and, if necessary, dying for the fatherland. Now, in our technologically advanced societies the aims of education appear to be social success, adaptation to a hierarchical system, integration into the great institutions that transform us into social creatures locked within the public services, and programmed preparation for adult life. It is as though education had become a productivity-linked investment in the future, a means of achieving economic goals. In socialist societies, the role of education is to diminish individualism, which suggests some kind of authoritarian conditioning. Those people who have been most receptive to Leboyer's 'marvellous poem to the glory of life and the joy in living' are almost certainly those who also listen enthusiastically to some of the progressive or alternative educationalists. The aim of life, they say, is the pursuit of happiness, the pursuit of an interest. The adult environment is not made for the child. True education must start by discovering the child so that it can be helped to accomplish its own liberation. Leboyer's ideas are the same as Maria Montessori's when she speaks of the 'intelligence of love' in the child, the intelligence that absorbs through love rather than indifference, by perceiving hidden qualities which only love can reveal. These are the ideas of Freinet, the ideas behind A. S. Neill's school Summerhill. Neill saw the child's role as being able to follow its own path, and not that conceived by anxious parents or advocated by educationalists. Adult interference or orientation of this kind can only produce a generation of robots. Here Neill and Leboyer are unanimous: neither will agree to manufacture automatons. But there is one important difference between them: like other educators Neill enters the life of the individual very much later than the obstetrician, and he knows it. His function is curative, to help children described as difficult because they are unhappy, in conflict with themselves and the rest of the world. Leboyer and Neill are seeking to create humanist socialism, socialism on a human scale, in which the individual can live without collective intervention, can find self-love without social anonymity, and take on the full extent of that freedom which our era has given us.

As we have seen, attempts to diminish the importance of birth can come from many sources, from doctors, sociologists, psychologists and educationalists. But whatever the source, none of them can devalue or alter the constructive thinking which Leboyer's work demands from us. Humankind is evolving in a vicious circle, but Leboyer has shown us a specific point at which we can take action. The nature of this vicious circle has been usefully described by Laborit (*Les Comportements*, 1973). Violence has facilitated the establishment of dominance in relations between individuals, groups of individuals and, above all, between nations. The dominant appear quite unaggressive because they maintain their position by means of a discreet institutionalized violence which is written into the prevailing ethical scale of values and prejudices; while the dominated have no other recourse than to an obvious actualized violence. The problem is to imagine a system in which the dominant human group can be included in an all-embracing whole without the opportunity either to dominate or to submit. On a world scale, when humankind is becoming a totality, there can be no question of force or revenge. Realistically speaking, we can only build a new world with the help of emotional energy, with love or the ability to love. But the ability to love is gradually becoming extinct, particularly in the dominant group, i.e. in the technologically advanced countries; and it is there that we should be working most urgently to give it new life. David Cooper's 'mourning black' is a color we should all be wearing:

> Why am I in mourning black?
> Mourning for the families I had
> for the madness I never had
> But now allow myself
> for the loss of love in the world. . .
> And I'm mourning over the death of
> love in the world
> And the non-distinction of death and love.
> I'm mourning about the non-distinction but also
> about an excess of distinctions.
> I'm mourning about my incapacity to
> break through all differentiations in the world
> so as to make the cosmos one activity . . .

In advanced industrial society there are many complementary factors contributing to the death of love. By considering the present conditions of birth, the early acquisition of the ability to love and to mother, and more especially the passing from one generation to the next of that ability, we are discovering and examining one of the most important cases of the death of love. More than that, we are able to see concrete solutions, to perceive a vulnerable point in the vicious circle. Obviously, the present conditions of birth are only one more symptom of the sickness threatening our civilization. In the world in which we live it is hardly surprising that newborn babies are received in the way they are. It is not unknown for the symptom to become pathogenic in itself. As Held said, 'Make us a better world and I will make you better mothers,' Aldous Huxley wrote, 'Give me better mothers and I will make you a better world.' There is no contradiction here, merely a germ of truth in both statements.

Perhaps, however, it is Huxley we should be listening to first, since he gives us a practical starting point. We must condemn the present conditions of birth. We must make a wider public aware.

Chapter Twelve
A CALL FOR MILITANCY

'The most important measure to be taken in the immediate present is to channel militant enthusiasm in an intelligent and responsible way, which means helping the younger generation to find causes worthy of service in our modern world.'
KONRAD LORENZ

How are we to raise the general consciousness and condemn the present conditions of birth? To whom should we be directing our words, and how?

Any attempt to create a new way of life (and like death, birth is another facet of our way of life), any attempt to change the system of human relations (and the mother-child relationship is only one specific case), any recreation of the great socialist dream of the utopians must rely on the kind of concerted militancy which can suggest an overall framework without falling permanently under the influence of those people who continue to demonstrate their sympathy and their desire to join the movement. This kind of militancy has proved effective in various fields during recent decades. The best example is the way in which we have managed to dissociate the two aspects of the sex act (and the resultant development of family planning). This is the best example, also, of liberation from the yoke imposed by nature or humanity. Some people have pointed to the contradiction between militancy, which implies fighting and struggle, and birth 'without violence'. But the kind of militancy we are talking about must be

recognized as merely a response to institutionalized
violence and a condemnation of the gratuitous violence
written into our traditions. The aim of our militant movement will not be to broadcast a system of concepts, but to
stimulate fresh thought about the present conditions of
birth in industrialized countries. The wide range of reasons
and arguments leading people to a shared awareness will
be the best surety against the formation of a group which
seeks to identify itself by a particular language or a
common conviction as distinct from the ignorant outsider.
To begin with, our effectiveness will depend on the degree
to which we can break down the barriers between the
world of the consumer and the world of the medical
professions. The humanization of hospitals is part of this
process.

The true importance of Leboyer's work can be seen in
relation to the new revolutionary movement. This movement is a direct response to the way in which the
structures of the industrial age have taken over our
society, depriving humans of all autonomy. The new
revolution will not be the product of armed struggle but
will be made in the body and soul of human beings. Illich
foresees a cultural and institutional revolution which will
restore humanity's control over its environment and will
lead ultimately to a convivial society in which humans
have mastery over the tools.

Something of this future revolution is evident in
Laborit's supposition that by suppressing the domination
instinct one would also suppress not only class struggles
but classes themselves. The essential factor in the evolution of a technological humanity would be the mental
restructuring of the greatest number of people, economic
alienation being only the consequence and not the cause

of intellectual and social alienation. The biologist in man, who immediately envisages the use of transforming and behavior-modifying drugs, takes no account of love, the origins of the ability to love and the way this is transmitted.

Gerard Mendel takes us a step further forward by introducing the concept of love and by stating that all forms of socialism which do not entail psychological modifications in the individual would appear doomed to failure. Self-love must no longer come through the intermediary of collectivity or idealization, but from ourselves as we take on all those freedoms which our time allows.

There were signs of this new revolutionary project in the traditional but now out-dated anarchism of the late 19th century which created theories to encompass certain manifestations of resistance to early industrial society. While simply a dream of traditional anarchism, this new project is central to modern anarchist activity. Anyone outside mainstream Marxism who still seeks a revolution will be trying to change life as a whole and will hear us; since changing life means first changing the way we are born.

More than anything else, Leboyer is a catalyst, perhaps even a mythical character. He has created a new language, a new code and it is to him that all future reference will have to be made whenever questions are asked about changing the conditions of birth in industrialized countries.

We join him in condemning the pride of the technician, in pointing to the dangers of an 'ethic of knowledge' of regarding the 'postulate of objectivity' as a condition of true knowledge. In our own way we too are imploring the elder not to hinder music.

In our convivial maternity unit we are constantly facing

experience and concept, constantly harmonizing the two. We have been granted the opportunity to move from an emotional awareness to a reasoned knowledge which has transformed our daily practice. In the terms of dialectical materialism, we have made a revolutionary leap forward.

Industrialized society is sinking into schizophrenia. Medicalized birth is speeding it along the way. There must be a new awareness, before Nemesis intervenes.

Recommended reading

As this edition is being printed for both the American and British markets, we list American and British publications separately:

USA

Ivan Illich *Medical Nemesis: The Expropriation of Health*, 1976, Pantheon
    Tools for Conviviality, 1973, Harper and Row
Sheila Kitzinger *The Experience of Breast-Feeding*, 1980 Penguin
    The Experience of Childbirth, 1972 Taplinger, 1978 Penguin
    Giving Birth: The Parents' Emotions in Childbirth, 1971, Taplinger, 1978 Schocken
    Women as Mothers: How they see themselves in different cultures, 1980, Random House
Marshall Klaus & John Kennell *Parent-Infant Bonding*, 1982, 2nd Ed., Mosby
Marshall Klaus & Martha Robertson *Birth, Interaction and Attachment*, 1983, Johnson and Johnson
Frederick Leboyer *Birth Without Violence*, 1975 Knopf
    Loving Hands: The Traditional Indian Art of Baby Massaging 1976, Stanford University Press

Great Britain

Ivan Illich *Limits to Medicine: Medical Nemesis, The Expropriation of Health*, 1976, Marion Boyars
    Tools for Conviviality, 1973, Marion Boyars

Sheila Kitzinger *Birth Over 30,* 1982, Sheldon Press
The Experience of Breast Feeding, 1979, Croom Helm
The Experience of Childbirth, 1962, Gollancz
Giving Birth: The Parents' Emotions in Childbirth, 1971, Sphere
New Good Birth Guide, 1983, Penguin
Marshall Klaus & John Kenell *Parent-Infant Bonding,* 1977 Mosby
Frederick Leboyer *Birth Without Violence,* 1975, Wildwood House

A Glossary for laymen

aspiration – the drawing in of air

cervical dilation (dilatation) – expansion of the neck of the womb

colitis – inflammation of the colon

electroencephalography – the science of electric brain measurements

endocrinology – the science of ductless glands which secrete hormones

ethnology – the science of human races, their relations and characteristics (anthropology)

ethology – the science of character formation and of animal behavior

eustachian tube – canal leading from the pharynx (muscles and membranes of nose, mouth and larynx) to the cavity of the tympanum (ear drum)

hypoglycemia – low blood sugar content

hyporeflexes – weak reflexes

hypothermia – low temperature

hypotonocity – weak muscle tones

hypotrophic – low weight

istrogenesis – disease caused by doctoring

occipitofrontal diameter – measures the back of the head to the forehead

olfactory – concerned with smelling

oncology – the science relating to tumors

pathogenesis – production or development of a disease

peritoneum – membrane which lines the cavity of the abdomen

prolactin – pituitary hormone which triggers off the secretion of milk

prophylaxis – the preventive treatment of disease
sacrum – a pelvic bone
sagittal diameter – measures distance between the right and left side of the skull
suture – the joining of the lips of a wound by stitches
vagus nerve – the pneumogastric (tenth cranial) nerve